The ObamaCare Reality

Is it really working?

Robert S. Roberts M.D.

ISBN: 1511937734
ISBN 13: 9781511937733

Also by Robert S. Roberts, M.D.

The ObamaCare Train Wreck

Dr. Bob's ObamaCare Blog
www.drbobroberts.com

Praise for *The ObamaCare Reality*

*"Every day, we see the harm ObamaCare is doing to American families and businesses. Folks are paying more and getting less, in the way of access to quality, affordable and innovative health care choices. In **The ObamaCare Reality**, Dr. Roberts presents a compelling case for how and why this is happening and why we need positive, patient-centered reforms to restore and protect the sacred doctor-patient relationship."*

U. S. Congressman Tom Price, M.D. (R – GA)
Chairman – House Budget Committee
Congressional Health Care Caucus

*"**The ObamaCare Reality** is informative, factual, and solution-based. Writing from a doctor's perspective, Dr. Roberts provides first-hand experience regarding the practical realities of the Affordable Care Act, as it passes its 5th anniversary and deepens its widespread impact on the American healthcare system."*

U. S. Congressman Daniel Webster (FL – 10)
House Committee on Transportation and Infrastructure

*"Dr. Roberts brings to **The ObamaCare Reality** the view of a surgeon who experiences government intrusion in our healthcare system everyday. He personally deals with the patients whose lives are being disrupted by the government takeover of what used to be the finest healthcare delivery system in the world. This book is a truthful account of ObamaCare, how it came about, how it is having such a negative effect on so many lives, and what the future looks like under this reformed effort."*

Florida Senator Alan Hays, DMD
Chairman – Appropriations Subcommittee on
General Government

Praise for *The ObamaCare Train Wreck*

*"**The ObamaCare Train Wreck** is a timely and very informative addition to the literature that attempts to preserve freedom and choice in America. It is a valuable resource for professionals and laymen alike and it makes sense!"*

> Benjamin S. Carson, Sr. M.D.
> New York Times Bestselling Author
> Professor Emeritus – Johns Hopkins Medical Center

*"**The ObamaCare Train Wreck** chronicles the road that led to a disaster in public policymaking and the fallout Americans all across the country are now facing. As more and more Americans discover the impact this will have on their lives, we are confronted with a sobering reminder of what's at stake in the fight to restore patient-centered health care."*

> Congressman Tom Price (Georgia – 06)
> Congressional Health Care Caucus
> Orthopedic Surgeon

"Dr. Roberts skillfully guides the reader through the fact and fiction of ObamaCare, including a point-by-point examination of the law's impact on physicians and their ability to meet the health care needs of their patients. His insights into what health care in America should be, and can be, are clearly stated and will be an important check list for future health care reform."

> Gary H. Mears
> Lt. General, USAF (Retired)

*"One of the greatest tragedies of the Affordable Care Act was the negligence of lawmakers to heavily consult the actual doctors and health care professionals outside of Washington who would be responsible for providing the services and navigating the added bureaucracy. A respected physician with years of experience, Dr. Roberts possesses a good grasp on the personal, practical, and political aspects of healthcare. **The ObamaCare Train Wreck** is a thoughtful manuscript that reveals some of the important factors that the White House did not take into account with their takeover of the federal health care system."*

> Congressman Daniel Webster (Florida – 10)

For Lois Ann, the best a man can get

Table of Contents

Introduction

"The usual suspects will keep crying failure, but the truth is that health reform is – gasp! – working."
Economist Paul Krugman, *The New York Times*, 7/13/14

People can be blinded by their ideology. It is a particular peculiarity of politics that those individuals with high intellects and even higher education can be especially immune to the most obvious observations of those of us with lesser intellectual gifts.

Case in point is Nobel-prize-winning economist Paul Krugman of Princeton University. Long known for his leftist ideology, Krugman is nevertheless a man of great intellect and education. How then to explain his complete misunderstanding of the real impact of ObamaCare?

As a regular columnist for *The New York Times*, Krugman has often written of his support for the Affordable Care Act. In a column entitled *ObamaCare Fails to Fail*, he asks a question that is pertinent:

"How many Americans know how health reform is going?"

Krugman accuses the American people of being ignorant of the many positive developments of the new healthcare law. Even more surprising, he accuses the media (never accused of right-wing bias) of even more ignorance, and failure to inform the public of the law's benefits. He laments the ACA thus: *"An immense policy success is improving the lives of millions of Americans, but it's largely slipping under the radar."*

Perhaps it is in defining success that there is room for disagreement. Krugman points to the initial debacle of the open enrollment period that eventually culminated in the enrollment of 7.1

million Americans (according to the White House) as a measure of success. But who expected such incompetence in simply developing an internet web site? This was never considered a principle objection of the law by those on the right who never voted for ObamaCare. To use a tennis term, it was an "unforced error" of the Obama administration. Solving this problem (and there is little evidence it has actually been solved) was never a measure of the success of the law itself.

Krugman claims a *"sharp reduction in the number of uninsured Americans"* but fails to remember that at least 6.2 million Americans, who had insurance before ObamaCare, lost their insurance as a direct result of the law. Even if you accept the numbers of newly enrolled being released by HHS Secretary Burwell, she still only claims 7 million enrolled at the start of the second open enrollment period – and only expects to reach a little over 9 million by 2015. Since the original goal was insuring 36 million more with ObamaCare, that's a long way from success by most peoples' standards.

To be sure, Krugman correctly points out that much of the increase in the number of insured has come in states that accepted the Medicaid expansion. He says, *"the decline in uninsured residents has been three times as large in Medicaid-expansion states as in Medicaid-expansion rejecters. It's not the economy; it's the policy, stupid."*

We'll discuss this liberal proclivity toward referring to the American people as "stupid" again in Chapter Fourteen. But before that, we'll discuss the wisdom of expanding Medicaid at all (Chapter Four), considering the quality of healthcare those unfortunate enough to be trapped in the Medicaid system must endure.

Krugman rightly asks why, if health reform is going so well, it continues to poll badly. His explanation is revealing:

"It's crucial, I'd argue, to realize that ObamaCare, by design, by and large doesn't affect Americans who already have good insurance. As a result, many peoples' views are shaped by the mainly negative coverage in the news media. Still, the latest tracking survey from the Kaiser Family Foundation shows that a rising number of Americans

are hearing about reform from family and friends, which means that they're starting to hear from the program's beneficiaries."

Let's analyze what he just said. First, he blames the bad poll numbers for ObamaCare on *"mainly negative coverage in the news media."* This is the first time in the Obama presidency years that I've heard that the problem with his policies is a hostile media. In fact, the opposite has been the case. Obama has enjoyed such a favorable media bias that Bernard Goldberg, long time respected journalist and TV newsman, wrote a book entitled *A Slobbering Love Affair: The Torrid Romance Between Barack Obama and the Mainstream Media.*

Second, he argues the latest tracking surveys from the Kaiser Family Foundation will somehow improve the healthcare law's standing in the polls. Yet he fails to reference the actual Kaiser poll numbers.

In reality, ObamaCare's popularity has *never* been good. In fact, when it was passed on March 23, 2010, polls showed more people opposed the law than supported it. At the time, House Majority Leader Nancy Pelosi assured us we'd love it as soon as we learned what was in it. She famously said, *"You have to pass the bill to find out what's in it."*

But it seems the more people find out what's in it *the less* they like it. New polls show the popularity of ObamaCare just keeps getting worse. According to *Real Clear Politics,* in Obama's second term alone, 140 polls have found ObamaCare to be unpopular. The number finding it to be popular? Zero.

Jeffrey H. Anderson, writing in *The Weekly Standard,* points out these 140 polls have shown that just 40 percent of Americans favor ObamaCare, while 52 percent oppose it. Of these 140 polls, 102 have shown double-digit deficits. Furthermore, *the trend is getting worse.* Since July 4 of 2014, all six polls taken have shown ObamaCare faring even worse with an average of 41 percent in favor but 55 percent opposed. In other words, the undecided are now coming down on the side of opposing ObamaCare while those who support it are about the same.

He also points out that *Real Clear Politics* didn't even include the notoriously left-leaning Kaiser Health Tracking Poll (the one Krugman cites). Yet even Kaiser has found ObamaCare to be unpopular in all

16 of its polls taken during Obama's second term. In these Kaiser polls only 37 percent favor the law while 53 percent oppose it.

Therefore, if you add the Kaiser polls to the rest you get 156 polls since the beginning of Obama's second term of office and *every single one shows more Americans oppose ObamaCare than support it*. There has not been a single poll showing more support than opposition to this healthcare law.

Professor Krugman is out of touch with reality. Even after the Democratic shellacking suffered in the November 2014 Mid-term elections, largely as a result of ObamaCare (Chapter 15), he still doubled-down on his defense of the law. But fortunately, the American people are beginning to learn the truth about ObamaCare.

Which brings me to the purpose of this book. My first book, *The ObamaCare Train Wreck,* chronicled the one hundred years history of healthcare reform beginning with the rise of the Progressives under President Theodore Roosevelt and culminating with the signing of the Patient Protection and Affordable Care Act (ObamaCare) on March 23, 2010, under President Barack Obama. The book then traces the implementation of the law through the end of the first open enrollment period, which closed on March 31, 2014.

This second book picks up where the first book ended, on April 1, 2014, and chronicles the changes that have taken place since then – and the experience of the American people actually living under the law. This book separates the fiction – as promoted by ObamaCare proponents like Krugman – from the reality of the law based on factual analysis.

It is not intended to be a criticism of liberal ideology, though by necessity it must address this issue at times, but rather an honest examination of the ObamaCare reality with the benefit now of one year's experience. All Americans deserve good healthcare – regardless of their ideological preference – and all Americans deserve the truth from their government. It is my hope that this book will help achieve both purposes.

Robert S. Roberts, M.D.
Orlando, Florida

1

The Premature Celebration

"The debate over repealing this law is over."
President Barack Obama – 4/1/14

The White House wanted to celebrate. Any excuse would do. April 1, 2014, marked the end of the open enrollment period for the Affordable Care Act, now widely known as ObamaCare. The new health care law, passed by Congress without a single Republican vote on March 23, 2010, had just completed its first open enrollment period that began on October 1, 2013.

The open enrollment period was an unmitigated disaster for the Obama White House from day one. Then HHS Secretary Kathleen Sebelius fended off criticism for the last six months because the government website, Healthcare.Gov, had failed repeatedly. After a start so appallingly bad that no one in the Obama administration would admit to the actual numbers enrolled, the White House was now feeling pretty good. (Recent information revealed now tells us only 6 people enrolled on the first day.)

As early as June, 2013, Secretary Sebelius was asked how many people needed to be enrolled by March 31, 2014, to consider the start a success. She repeatedly came up with the number 7 million which she called "a realistic target". But not long after the abysmal start of October, 2013, she was trying to push back from that number.

Vice-President Joe Biden modified the expectations of the White House to "5 or 6 million," calling this a success. Sebelius was then asked about this remark in a *Huffington Post* interview with progressive commentator Marc Lamont Hill. She responded that the White House never considered the seven million number to be a benchmark of success. She said, *"First of all, seven million was not the administration. That was a CBO, Congressional Budget Office, prediction when the bill was first signed. I'm not sure where they even got their numbers."*

Rose Garden Ceremony

Yet, somehow when the dust settled on March 31, the White House was gleefully announcing that *"7.1 million have signed-up."* President Obama was quick to announce these unexpected numbers in a Rose Garden ceremony on April 1st. Suddenly all the angst about ObamaCare was gone and liberals were declaring victory.

The *Wall Street Journal* editorial board was skeptical, declaring,

"The government appears to have tapped heretofore-unknown reserves of bureaucratic efficiency by releasing numbers timed to this campaign-style rally. Yet for months the Health and Human Services Department has refused to disclose crucial contextual data, such as how many insurance contracts are in force, the market-by-market totals and how many beneficiaries were previously covered. Regardless of your partisan sympathies the White House's selective disclosure is a crime against transparency and accountable government."

But Obama's rhetoric was nevertheless soaring. *"The Affordable Care Act is here to stay,"* he declared. *"The bottom line is this: Under this law, the share of Americans with insurance is up, and the growth of health care costs is down. And that's good for our middle class, and that's good for our fiscal future. . . . The debate over repealing this law is over."*

The president is fond of saying, *"the debate is over."* He used the same phrase in his 2014 State of the Union address when referring to global warming. Yet climate data are inconveniently not cooperating with this analysis. The last seventeen years have recorded global cooling and there is recent evidence the polar ice cap is actually getting larger. Perhaps when you're losing the debate it's time to declare it is over.

In fact, liberals are having a hard time getting anyone to take their global warming theories seriously, anymore. On September 23, 2014, the United Nations hosted an event for world leaders in New York City to discuss urgent action they believe is needed against climate change. Yet the leaders of China, India, and Germany decided to skip the event. It seems no one is buying the U. N.'s concerns.

But who could blame them? Even the United Nations' own Intergovernmental Panel on Climate Change no longer claims there will be dangerous or rapid climate change in the next two decades. They downgraded their usual alarmist forecast to predict the global warming will amount to a mere O.5 degrees Celsius (0.9 degrees Fahrenheit) over the next 30 years.

Matt Ridley, writing in *The Wall Street Journal,* thinks even that prediction is likely too high. He reminds us that global warming actually stopped about 17 years ago. He writes, *"First the climate-research establishment denied that a pause existed, noting that if there was a pause, it would invalidate their theories. Now they say there is a pause (or "hiatus") but that it doesn't after all invalidate their theories. Alas, their explanations have made their predicament worse by implying that man-made climate change is so slow and tentative that it can be easily overwhelmed by natural variation in temperature – a possibility that they had previously all but ruled out."*

This book is not intended as a rebuttal on the issue of climate change, but it is worth noting that President Obama has a habit of trying to cut off debate when facts get in the way of his rhetoric. We will see how this applies often to the issue of healthcare reform.

White House Spin
It was no surprise then that the White House declared they had 7.1 million Americans "signed up." You had to know they would announce

this success even though they could not give us any details regarding how many of these had actually paid for their insurance, how many represented newly insured Americans as opposed to those whose policies were cancelled due to ObamaCare, or any of the demographic breakdown details regarding age or pre-existing medical conditions.

We know that 6.2 million Americans or more lost their health insurance policies in 2013 when their insurance companies were forced to cancel policies that failed to comply with the stringent new standards of ObamaCare. (The number would have been much higher if the Employer Mandate had not been delayed by President Obama.) So the 7.1 million new "sign ups" might actually only represent 900 thousand newly insured Americans when those who lost their insurance due to the law are counted.

But even that assumes all of these people have actually purchased a policy. The reports from insurance industry insiders say at least 20 percent of the "sign ups" failed to make a payment so the real number of insured was probably at least 20 percent lower. That brings the number of newly insured down to about 720 thousand.

Nevertheless, Democrats were suddenly invigorated. Those Senators up for re-election in Red states believed they were reborn. Instead of running from their voting record on ObamaCare they suddenly were willing to double down on their rhetoric. Louisiana's Mary Landrieu said ObamaCare *"holds great promise and is getting stronger every day."* Alaska's Mark Begich declared *"seven million people have access to quality, affordable care and are in control of their own health-care choices."* House Minority Leader Nancy Pelosi boasts Congressional Democrats *"are happy to not run away from what we have done. We're very proud of what we have accomplished."*

Republicans Encouraged

Republicans were happy the Democrats were so proud. (*"Pride goes before destruction, and haughtiness before a fall." - Proverbs 16:18)*. Already the Republicans won a pivotal test of the impact of ObamaCare when Republican David Jolly of Florida defeated

Democratic favorite Alex Sink in a special election to fill a vacant House seat. Despite Democratic claims to the contrary, it is clear that ObamaCare played a big role in altering the outcome of that race that many had conceded to the Democrats.

Karl Rove, former deputy chief of staff for President George W. Bush, writing in *The Wall Street Journal* said, *"ObamaCare is and will remain a political problem for Democrats because there's a huge disconnect between the party's rhetoric and the reality that people affected by the law have experienced. . . Even if the administration gets seven million paying customers on the exchanges, they can't assume they are all happy patrons who will vote Democratic in gratitude. Most are people whose health coverage was canceled last fall despite Mr. Obama's frequent promise that "if you like your plan, you can keep your plan."*

Remember that those who lost their plans had chosen those plans on their own and most were happy with them. Now they had new plans with mandated greater coverage for treatments many do not need such as maternity coverage for men and contraceptives for nuns.

Many are paying more for that unwanted additional coverage, especially young people who are being compelled to subsidize the costs of older, sicker Americans. Many have lost their doctor, who is not available on the exchanges, because provider fees have been lowered. It is unlikely these people will feel the love for the Democrats that made them purchase these unwanted policies and caused them to lose their doctor.

But all of this was speculation on April 1, 2014. While the White House was celebrating, the real issue was not how many people may or may not be enrolled in ObamaCare but how many people are getting the healthcare they need. The failures of the Obama administration to build a successful website for purchasing insurance were never expected. No one predicted the disastrous rollout of the new healthcare law in the criticism that followed the law's passage in 2010.

The real concern is how well will the law succeed in meeting its goals. Will the law provide the increased insurance coverage for those Americans currently uninsured? *Will the insurance they receive actually result in better healthcare?* Behind all the rhetoric on both sides of the aisle, the issue should be about providing the best healthcare for all Americans. Isn't that what the law was supposed to provide?

State v. Federal Exchanges

To answer these and many other questions about how well the law is working, we must look at what is actually happening. We must go beyond the spin of the White House to get the truth behind their press releases. We must find out how real Americans are receiving their health care.

First, let's look at the insurance exchanges set up by the state and federal governments. The Affordable Care Act proposed that every state set up its own insurance exchange to sell state residents the new health insurance. The federal government would also set up an exchange that would handle all those states that chose not to participate. Unfortunately for the Obama administration, 36 of the 50 states refused to set up their own exchange.

This was particularly alarming to the White House since subsidies for lower income Americans were only permitted by the law if purchased on a state exchange. This meant all those individuals purchasing their health insurance on the federal exchange were ineligible for subsidies. We will discuss this in more detail in Chapter Two, but the White House chose to ignore the law and provide subsidies for everyone, even on the federal exchange.

In the fourteen states and the District of Columbia where they did set up their own exchanges, most of them have been a disaster. Much like the federal exchange, these states have had great difficulty building websites that can perform all of the necessary functions required by this law.

The problem is verification of income. In order for people to be eligible for subsidies, the government must verify their income. This requires links between the government website and the

IRS. Furthermore, they must verify identification, immigration and employment status. They must do all of this in a secure environment lest identity thieves steal the information for their own criminal purposes. All of these functions proved to be too cumbersome for most of the state and federal exchanges.

Ironically, many of the states scrambling to come up with a working state exchange are deeply blue states that supported President Obama's election and are led by governors that supported passage of the Affordable Care Act. Not surprisingly, all of them supported Medicaid expansion under the new law. These seven liberal states, Oregon, Massachusetts, Maryland, Minnesota, Nevada, Vermont, and Hawaii, have state exchanges that have either completely failed or are on life support.

In order to prevent such failures, the Centers for Medicaid and Medicare Services (CMS) established "gate reviews" to monitor progress in the development of state insurance exchanges. These "gate reviews" were periodic assessments of progress in seven areas. Successful completion of these reviews enabled states to continue receiving federal funds for the process. Despite these reviews, and continued funding, these states failed anyway.

Oregon

These failures have come at great expense to the taxpayers. Oregon has spent over $300 million so far on their *Cover Oregon* web site and has yet to enroll anyone except by paper applications. After repeated complaints by a state representative, the FBI, the HHS inspector general, and the Government Accountability Office (GAO) have launched investigations into whether or not state officials misrepresented their progress in order to keep their funding. There is some evidence to suggest the web site was never intended to function; a fake web site. If true, this would represent criminal activity.

The state has struggled to keep up with the demand for new enrollees by filling out over 300,000 applications by paper. But with no hope of solving the state exchange problems before the next enrollment period in November, state officials turned to the federal government's Healthcare.gov web site. According to *The Wall Street Journal,* the cost of migrating to the federal exchange will be another $41 million.

Maryland

The situation in Maryland is similar. Although it was one of the first states to begin building its exchange, the web site crashed just after the October 1 launch. The state brought in United Health Group in December to fix the website well enough for the open-enrollment period but it continued to suffer failures. The state finally voted to scrap the website and start over with the system used by the more successful Connecticut exchange. Over 290,000 applications were completed by hand to meet the demand for new enrollees. The state has already spent another $300 million taxpayer dollars and will need about $50 million more to fix the problems.

Michael Astrue, former commissioner of Social Security and general counsel of the U.S. Department of Health and Human Services, has placed the blame for this fiasco at the feet of HHS Inspector General Daniel Levinson. He first called attention to this problem in October 2013, in *The Weekly Standard,* and then wrote an update later called *ObamaCare in the Blue States.*

He called for an investigation of Maryland, similar to that presently being conducted in Oregon, by the FBI and HHS Inspector General Levinson. This will be an early test of new HHS Secretary Sylvia Mathews Burwell, who has already pledged to use "the full extent of the law" to recover misspent health exchange funding. If she fails to pursue an investigation of Maryland we can expect much of the same foot-dragging that characterized the tenure of her predecessor.

Massachusetts – home of RomneyCare

Perhaps no state was expected to have a more seamless transition to the new healthcare law than Massachusetts. The state was already the poster-child for a similar healthcare plan dubbed "RomneyCare" after Governor Mitt Romney, who presided over its implementation. *The Connector*, as it is called, has been in use since 2006.

But conversion of the state to the new ObamaCare plan proved more difficult than expected. Even now the state exchange still does not allow residents to obtain insurance as the ACA requires. State officials are currently debating whether or not to rebuild the website or convert to Healthcare.gov. Some have estimated the state has already spent $135 million and expect the cost of conversion to reach $121 million more. Others say the true figure is over half a billion dollars.

Governor Duval Patrick has impeded attempts by his Democratic legislature to obtain an accounting of where the money has gone. As part of his response to the crisis, Patrick has placed as many as 200,000 applicants, who requested financial assistance, on Medicaid – whether they qualified for Medicaid or not. This means additional expense to the taxpayers for payments made by Medicaid for ineligible patients. Again, the question is, "Where is CMS and where is the inspector general?"

Minnesota

The same sorry scenario played out in Minnesota as well. Once again, state officials appear to have withheld important information from the state board, the public, and the insurance companies, needed to implement the system. The *MNsure* website collapsed despite the fact that they were able to pass the CMS "gate reviews".

The real question is how did states like these slip through the process of "gate reviews" and continue to receive federal funding of non-functioning exchanges?

Astrue complains, *"Again, ill-advised software contracts compounded timeline failures produced primarily by poor planning and execution. Somehow, Minnesota also miraculously passed the CMS gate reviews even though, as in Massachusetts, it could not test a beta system before its failed launch. We need to know how CMS could have possibly found adequate progress for functionality and security in light of this disarray, and law enforcement needs to know too."*

Nevada

The situation is not much better in Nevada, home of then-Senate Majority Leader Harry Reid. They extended the period of enrollment all the way to the end of May to allow those affected by technical glitches to complete their enrollment. The Nevada Association of Health Plans said insurance carriers are receiving incorrect payment and enrollment information and they are concerned that people may be terminated from their plans for non-payment.

A class-action lawsuit was filed in May against the state's exchange and contractor Xerox on behalf of Nevada residents who say they've paid their premiums but don't have insurance. On May 20 the state announced their decision to shut down their state exchange and convert to Healthcare.gov for at least a year.

Hawaii

Hawaii suffers from low enrollment numbers, just like these other states. This threatens the long-term stability of its exchange. They have enrolled 7,200 in private plans and have a backlog of 11,000 applications needing to be processed. They already had a low number of uninsured residents prior to the ACA since a 1974 law that required most employers to provide coverage to employees who work more than 20 hours per week. (The ACA only requires this of employees working 30 or more hours per week.)

Vermont

Vermont, home of openly socialist Senator Bernie Sanders, still faces enormous problems implementing ObamaCare despite its tiny population. Sanders has often expressed his preference for a single-payer system much like Canada. The state used the same vendor, CGI, that failed so spectacularly in implementing the federal website and gave them until July 2 to get the site working. It is not clear what they will do if CGI fails again.

Seven states; four with completely failed exchanges and three on life support. Thus far the cost of government ineptness in just these states has been over $1.2 billion dollars ($1,279,033,737 according to CMS) with another $240 million estimated future expenses to fix the problems, according to sources at *The Wall Street Journal.* Two important dates loomed as these states struggled to provide functioning exchanges; First, the November 15, 2014 date for open enrollment; Second, the January 1, 2015 date when HHS loses authority to issue grants to states for their exchanges.

It is no surprise that those states that are dominated by liberal politicians are quick to spend the taxpayers' money. Yet it is curious that those most in favor of instituting government control of healthcare seem least capable of implementing it. This bodes poorly for the future of ObamaCare.

Will the voters hold their elected officials accountable for this inept and wasteful start? It seems unlikely in blue states that voters will change their opinions nor acknowledge the futility of this government takeover of health care. But voters' opinions may change quickly when their own healthcare is at stake. Loyalty to party may be trumped by the need to find the right doctor in times of crisis. The results of the November, 2014 mid-term elections showed how the voters decided. (Chapter 15)

The Effectiveness of the Enrollment

Beyond the issue of the cost of enrollment is the larger issue of the number of Americans actually enrolled. The primary purpose of the Affordable Care Act was to increase the number of insured Americans.

How effective has the enrollment been in accomplishing this primary purpose? Not very good, it seems.

At the end of the open enrollment on March 31, 2014, the White House announced that 7.1 million Americans had enrolled in ObamaCare. They increased that number shortly thereafter to 8.0 million. The liberal *Los Angeles Times* went so far as to call the number

9.5 million based on an as-yet-unpublished RAND Corporation survey. The assumption in these figures was that all of these people were previously uninsured and their new coverage was attributable to ObamaCare. But clearly this was wishful thinking.

Chris Conover, writing in *Forbes* did a careful analysis of the *Los Angeles Times* estimate. He summarizes his findings thus:

- **Hard Truth #1 – The total number of uninsured has NOT declined by 9.5 million**

  The *LA Times* figure assumes 2 million uninsured purportedly covered through the Exchanges, 3 million previously uninsured young adults purportedly covered under their parents' policies, and 4.5 million covered through **Medicaid**.

  Conover says the *L A Times* itself reports, "*Fewer than a million people who had health plans in 2013 are now uninsured because their plans were cancelled for not meeting new standards set by the law, the RAND survey indicates.*" That means we must subtract ~ 1 million newly uninsured from the 9.5 million with gives us now 8.5 million.

  Furthermore, *the number of previously uninsured young adults covered by parents is half as large as reported.* The originally reported number was 3.1 million based on an analysis of data from the National Health Interview Survey. Since then, two much larger surveys both show much smaller declines: 1.8 million according to the American Community Survey (ACS) and 1.4 million using the Current Population Survey (CPS). Conover splits the difference and estimates 1.6 million fewer uninsured young adults due to parental coverage. That lowers the net reduction number to **7.1 million.**

- **Hard Truth #2 – Performance is well below CBO projections**

  The Congressional Budget Office (CBO) is considered non-partisan and has been the "official scorekeeper" for ObamaCare since its inception.

The CBO has varied its projections since March 2010 when the law was first passed. The original chart showed 59.3 % reduction in March 2010 but has since been revised to 37.3 % as seen in Figure One below. This original estimate expected nearly a two-fifths reduction by 2014 alone. (All estimates shown are calculated by comparing CBO's projection of the reduction in the number of uninsured under the law to its projection for the number of uninsured in 2014 without the law.) In less than a year they had to lower expectations to under 40%.

Expectations continued to decline over time, especially after the June 2012 Supreme Court decision which gave states the right to decide for themselves whether or not to expand Medicaid eligibility under the law. In February 2014 they had lowered their projections to under 23%. At the time of the close of the enrollment period on March 31, 2014, the actual numbers were only 12.5%. (Figure 1)

Despite declining CBO expectations, the actual reduction in uninsured Americans is about half of CBO projections for 2014

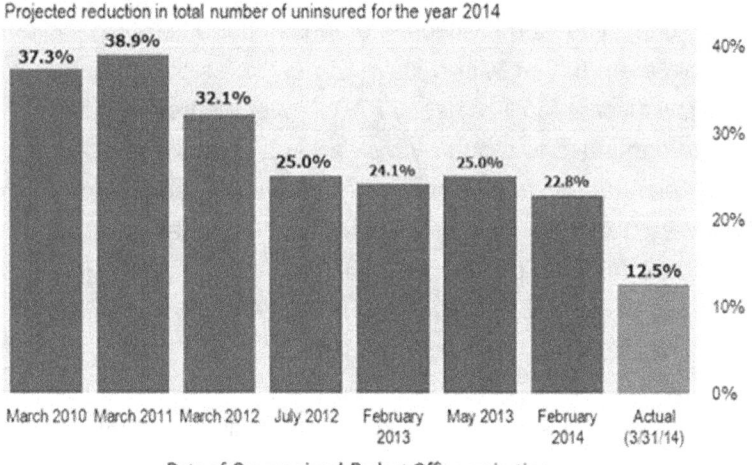

Projected reduction in total number of uninsured for the year 2014

Date of Congressional Budget Office projection

Figure 1 – CBO projections from March 2010 through 3/31/14.

What should we expect going forward? The numbers will probably decline since many people will fail to keep up their insurance premium payments. Robert Laszewski, health insurance industry expert, reports about 2-5% of those who enrolled have never paid their second premium. If they continue to fail to make payments they will be dropped from the rolls of those with insurance coverage.

There are other problems, too. Many of those who enrolled received subsidies; in fact about 87% according to insurance industry reports. Those subsidies are predicated on income information supplied at the time of enrollment. Due to the failures of the government web site Healthcare.gov, this income information could not be verified at the time of enrollment. Over a million people have been asked for additional information to verify their income. If they fail to provide income verification, they will also lose their coverage.

- **Likely Truth #3 – Had CBO projections been accurate, ObamaCare never would have passed**

Conover's analysis is that we have expanded coverage to 1 in 8 uninsured Americans. But at the same time, we have disrupted coverage for millions, increased premiums for tens of millions more, and amplified the pain even further with a wave of new taxes and fees that will cost even low income families nearly $7,000 over the next decade.

He continues to stand by his earlier analysis (reported in my first book *The ObamaCare Train Wreck*) that we will see **at least 4 "losers" for every "winner" under ObamaCare,** especially given that nearly two thirds (4.5 million of the 7.1 million) of the newly insured have gained their coverage through Medicaid rather than private insurance. Was it worth this?

Imagine if Congress had known the following facts before they voted for the law in March, 2010:

- **12.5% fewer uninsured by 2014 rather than 37.3%**

- **Millions with cancelled coverage, of which 1 million remain uninsured**
- **A $2 *trillion* increase in the federal debt in its first two decades rather than a deficit reduction**
- **Far higher premium increase in the non-group, small group and large group markets than originally estimated**
- **Nearly $7,000 in added taxes/fees over a decade even for families in the lowest 20% of household income**

As it was, the law was passed without a single Republican vote. However, if the above facts were known at the time of the vote, surely some of the Democratic members of Congress would have objected as well.

Perhaps you think Conover's analysis is too harsh. It can actually be argued he was too conservative. Glenn Kessler, fact-checker at *The Washington Post,* dug into the RAND survey numbers further. He found the Medicaid figure showed an increase from 7.7% in 2013 to 10% in 2014; but this survey had a margin of error of 2 points so the actual number could have been 8 or 12%. The *LA Times* calculated the increase at 4.5 million. With the margin of error at 2% the actual numbers could swing dramatically in either direction.

There are other issues for those who wish to dig deeper. First, not every new Medicaid enrollee would have been previously uninsured. The RAND survey doesn't answer that question. They estimate that of 13.1 million net new Medicaid enrollees in 2016, 10.8 million (82%) would come from the ranks of the previously uninsured. So if 82% of the estimated 4.5 million added to Medicaid are uninsured, then the net reduction in uninsured ranks would be 3.7 million. This further reduces the 7.1 million number to now only 6.3 million.

Second, there is the "what would have happened otherwise" issue. If you look at the trend for Medicaid enrollment figures prior to passage of ObamaCare you will see enrollment was growing as a share of the non-elderly population. According to the American

Community Survey, those numbers would have been 17.8% in 2012 vs. 16.9% in 2010; a 5.3% increase in chances of being on Medicaid. If this is so, another 5.3% of the reduction in the uninsured should be subtracted from the number, which brings it down to about 6.1 million.

Kessler correctly points out that even at 4.5 million for the number of newly enrolled Medicaid, this figure is only slightly over half of the 8 million projected by CBO in February 2014. *Is the glass half-empty or half-full?*

A More Recent Analysis

Perhaps you think the analysis of Chris Conover was premature. His article was written in April 2014, just after the end of the open enrollment for ObamaCare. Things might have gotten better.

Jeffrey H. Anderson, writing in *The Weekly Standard,* updates our information. In July 2014 he wrote:

"In March 2010, ObamaCare was about to be voted upon by the House of Representatives, and the Democrats were in the process of deciding whether to ignore public opinion at their peril. At that time, the CBO projected that ObamaCare would cost $938 Billion over a decade and would reduce the number of uninsured people by 19 million as of 2014 (with a reduction of 1 million prior to 2014 and 18 million in 2014 alone). . . .

Now the Urban Institute finds that ObamaCare has actually reduced the number of uninsured adults by 8 million since the rollout began last fall. (Gallop shows a similar number.) That's far short of the number of newly insured that the CBO projected in April of this year, in February of this year, or in 2012 – and it's less than half the tally the American people were told ObamaCare would hit when they opposed it in 2010."

This analysis also indicates the CBO predictions of February 2014 were optimistic, at best.

Even the White House is now adjusting their numbers downward. As of September 19, they reduced their ObamaCare enrollment number to 7.3 million. (In November the number was down to 7.1 million). Naturally, they did not release any details regarding the breakdown of this number. The number was described in a *Politico* article thus:

"The figure is complex to unravel. The number came from the health insurers, who told the Obama administration every month how many people are covered by Affordable Care Act plans. A CMS official said Thursday that in prior monthly reports, the numbers varied widely, but recently stabilized."

Insurance industry expert Robert Laszewski analyzed this recent statement with the following comments:

"So this tells us a couple of things:

1. *The carriers have been reporting the number of people they have been insuring in the exchanges to the Obama administration for months.*
2. *The monthly enrollment numbers have "varied widely."*

Up until now, the administration has repeatedly said they didn't have the enrollment numbers. Why haven't they released these monthly reports on an ongoing basis? Why can't we see all of the prior reports?"

The 7.3 million-enrollment number would seem to suggest only a 9% attrition factor when most carriers have been reporting that about 15% haven't paid just the first premium. Even with the lack of transparency about just what these numbers mean, I can find at least one obvious problem with them.

As I thought of the administration's release of 7.3 million it occurred to me that they said the 7.3 million included all enrollments through mid-August. Under ObamaCare, after a person has paid their first premium, a health plan can't cancel anyone until they have gone three months without making a payment. So, they are effectively double counting by including the "adds' while also keeping the "deletes".

The 7.3 million figure includes all of the enrollments that have occurred through mid-August. But the number also still includes every person who has failed to make a premium payment in June, July, and August – since the carriers can't yet knock them off the rolls. The health plans tell me there is a 2% to 4% monthly attrition rate. That means the 7.3 million could be overstated by 6 to 12% of the total."

So even when the White House is trying to give us more reasonable enrollment numbers, they still fudge them. If Laszewski is correct, the real numbers, even using the White House figure, is somewhere between 6 % lower, or 6.8 million, or even 12% lower, or 6.4 million. That raises the obvious question as to how these numbers compare to the number of uninsured before ObamaCare.

The Uninsured Before ObamaCare

In 2010, before ObamaCare, there were about 50 million people or 16% of the population in America without health insurance. Of these about 13 million were illegal aliens that never qualified for ObamaCare insurance. So about 37 million were uninsured and eligible for ObamaCare.

President Obama campaigned for the presidency by promising, *"I will sign a universal health care bill into law by the end of my first term as president that will cover every American."* (June 23, 2007).

The best estimates of the architects of ObamaCare predicted the new law would cover about 95 % of the population with the only remaining uninsured being illegal aliens, those who refused to purchase insurance, or those eligible for Medicaid who failed to enroll; a number estimated at about 17 million or 5 % of the population.

However, in 2014 the CBO revised their earlier projections and now expect by 2024 there will still be about 31 million uninsured Americans or about 10% of the population. By those estimates, the new health care law only improves coverage of the uninsured by 19 million or about 6% of the population.

But now come estimates that predict the number of uninsured Americans who are not illegal aliens will be 40 million by 2024. That's about 10% more than the 37 million who were uninsured when the law was passed in 2010. In an article published in *The Wall Street Journal,* authors Stephen T. Parente and Bianca Frogner explain their reasoning. Parente is associate dean of the Carlson School of Management and director of the Medical Industry Leadership Institute at the University of Minnesota and Frogner is a professor at George Washington University.

They see that rising premium costs and out-of-pocket expenses will force low to middle income consumers out of the private insurance market. They estimate average premiums on the individual exchange health plan (Silver) will increase by $1,375 by 2019 while the average family premium for the same plan will increase by $2,198 – outpacing the average increases from 2008 to 2013. The steepest increase in these prices will be seen in 2017 for three reasons:

- All plans, including those currently exempt for hardship and old plans extended for various reasons – **must comply with the "essential health benefits" rules** enacted by the HHS Secretary. As many as 60% of plans sold in 2013 were non-compliant.
- The "**reinsurance program**" will expire in 2017, meaning health insurers will no longer be reimbursed by the government for their uncovered expenses.
- The "**risk corridors**" program will also expire in 2017. (Chapter Five) The insurance companies will look now to consumers, rather than the government, to pick up the tab for these high cost policies.

Don't expect government subsidies to keep up with these sharply rising premium expenses.

Consumers will be forced into one of several poor options. Purchase lower cost high-deductible plans and hope they don't have to use them; sign up for Medicaid if they're eligible, or go without insurance at all. The loss of these individuals from the private insurance market will drive up premiums even higher for those who continue to purchase their insurance. This may further increase the number who refuse to purchase insurance, creating an insurance "death spiral".

The Impact of ObamaCare

Parente and Frogner predict over 5 million will lose their employer-provided insurance as employers favor letting employees get their insurance on the exchanges. The CBO has actually estimated this number at 7 million by 2020. They believe Medicaid enrollment will increase by 2-3% annually through 2024. But many will not be eligible for the program, especially since half of the states decided not to expand Medicaid under ObamaCare because of fears of rising state expenses.

The result of these changes will be many uninsured Americans who will accept the government tax for failure to purchase insurance; $695 or 2.5% of income, whichever is greater, after 2016. By their calculations, this will leave 40 million Americans uninsured by 2024, not counting illegal aliens.

If their calculations are correct, this means after 10 years of ObamaCare there will be about *10% more Americans uninsured than before the law was enacted!* After trillions of your tax dollars have been spent by the government to provide insurance for those currently uninsured, there will actually be more Americans uninsured. *This exposes ObamaCare for what it really is: a government takeover of healthcare for the purposes of control and redistribution of wealth.*

Parente concludes,

*"So perishes the Affordable Care Act's promise to deliver universal health care – its fatal conceit. The autopsy will show that it died from a lack of affordability, leaving behind millions of Americans who were sold a bill of goods. **One thing is painfully clear: that isn't what the doctor ordered."***

Second Enrollment Numbers

The second open enrollment of ObamaCare ended on February 15th. According to HHS Secretary Burwell everything is going great.

President Obama goes so far to say, *"The Affordable Care Act is working. It's working a little better than we expected."*

Laszewski's predictions for the second open enrollment period warned that enrollment numbers could not be trusted for at least 90 days after the end of enrollment. That's because the insurance industry cannot drop the policies of previous policyholders for 90 days even after they fail to make a payment. The result will be many duplications when counting new enrollment.

With the close of the second open enrollment, the White House claimed 11.4 million people signed up for ObamaCare. Laszewski says the actual number will drop to about 10.5 million based upon his conversations with the insurance industry. But even if he concedes as many as 11 million enrolled, would that exceed expectations?

Table 1 shows the Congressional Budget Office (CBO) projections for enrollment in May 2013. These projections were decreased from earlier projections and intended to portray a more accurate representation of expectations.

Table 1. CBO's May 2013 Estimate of the Effects of the Affordable Care Act on Health Insurance

EFFECTS ON INSURANCE COVERAGE[a]		2013	2014	2015	2016	2017	2018
(Millions of nonelderly people, by calendar year)							
Prior-Law Coverage[b]	Medicaid and CHIP	35	34	34	33	33	33
	Employment-Based	156	157	159	161	164	165
	Nongroup and Other[c]	25	25	26	26	27	27
	Uninsured[d]	57	57	57	56	56	55
	TOTAL	272	274	276	277	279	281
Change	Medicaid and CHIP	1	9	12	12	12	12
	Employment-Based[e]	2	*	-2	-6	-6	-7
	Nongroup and Other[c]	*	-2	-3	-4	-5	-5
	Insurance Exchanges	0	7	13	22	24	25
	Uninsured[d]	-2	-14	-20	-25	-25	-25
Uninsured Under the Affordable Care Act							
Number of Uninsured Nonelderly People[d]		55	44	37	31	30	30
Insured Share of the Nonelderly Population[e]							
Including All Residents		80%	84%	86%	89%	89%	89%
Excluding Unauthorized Immigrants		82%	86%	89%	91%	92%	92%

The table may seem confusing but the message is that the CBO estimated in 2013 that there would be an average of 13 million people in the insurance exchanges during 2015. Recalling the first open enrollment that ended April 1, 2014, the White House claimed 7.1 million enrolled, then 8 million, but eventually conceded that number dropped to 6.7 million by the end of 2014. A similar attrition would take an 11 million enrollment to about 9 million by the end of 2015. The HHS own 2015 estimate is for 9.1 million.

Next, remember the CBOs original enrollment projection for 2016 was 22 million. So, at the end of 2014 they had 6.7 million, at the end of 2015 they will likely have 9 million. Is 22 million a realistic number for 2016?

Why This Matters

Perhaps you're thinking this is "much ado about nothing." Why do all these numbers matter?

The primary purpose of the Affordable Care Act was to insure the uninsured. President Obama famously claimed in 2007 he would *"cover every American"* with health insurance. But the CBO, which has missed its projections every time so far, still projects 31 million Americans will be uninsured by 2016. If their projections continue to be overly optimistic, as they have been in the past, the number of uninsured by 2016 may approach 40 million. This is only slightly less than the number of uninsured before the law was passed!

Laszewski offers insurance industry insider knowledge that explains other reasons it matters. He says ObamaCare needs to have a sustainable population participating by the time the insurance company support (the 3Rs of the insurance bailout provisions of the law) expires at the end of 2016. The long-time insurance industry-underwriting rule is that you need 75% of an eligible group to be confident of a sustainable risk pool.

By this standard, they will need to enroll 75% of the 17.2 million eligible for enrollment by the end of 2016. That means their goal should be 12.9 million by 2016. Shooting for only 9 to 9.9 million this year seems like a low number and will put much more pressure on the administration in 2016.

It also matters because rising numbers of uninsured create political pressure to do something better. It matters financially because uninsured people raise the cost of insurance premiums for those who actually pay for them. That means premium prices go up for everyone.

Lastly, Laszewski warns us that the "back room" of Healthcare.gov is still not completely built. That means the web site can't pay the insurance companies. Insurers are still getting paid based upon a workaround that involves them manually filing out worksheets – for 7 million people.

Healthcare.gov also can't reconcile the cost sharing subsidies the lowest income people get from ObamaCare – like lower deductibles and co-pays. This increases the inaccuracy of the enrollment numbers. Laszewski reports one insurance carrier told him they only ended up with half of the net January enrollments the web site originally reported to them.

President Obama claims, *"It's working a little better than expected."* This is clearly a political, even delusional statement. Unless enrollment numbers greatly improve in the next two years, ObamaCare will be unable to sustain itself with affordable insurance premiums. The dire predictions of Parente and Frogner that there will still be 40 million uninsured Americans by 2024 may well come true.

Therefore, it is apparent at this writing, the primary goal of ObamaCare to greatly increase the number of Americans with health insurance will fail to materialize. This was actually the most achievable goal. We will see how other goals will fail more dramatically - with more costly consequences.

2

The Impact of Judicial Decisions

"It is not our job to protect the people from the consequences of their political choices."
U.S. Supreme Court Chief Justice John Roberts – 6/30/12

Criticism of the majority party in office is nothing new in this country. Indeed, it is a vital part of our democracy and should it ever cease, so too would our freedom.

Yet, it is also inherent in our democracy that those in office seek compromise with those in the minority party lest the people believe they are being bludgeoned by the majority. History is replete with revolutions that broke out when the minority felt so mistreated. Our own country was formed from such turmoil, and the revolutions of France and Russia also testify to the dangers of political over-reach.

Therefore, those who have studied this history must have been concerned when the Obama administration and the Democratic Party bludgeoned the Republicans by passing ObamaCare without a single Republican vote. Never in the history of this country has the majority party passed such monumental legislation on completely partisan lines.

President Obama achieved this singular legislative victory at great expense. This unilateral action drew a line in the sand that guaranteed challenges in the judicial system and assured even stiffer opposition by Republicans of any future legislation. In this chapter I will review the key judicial challenges to ObamaCare and how they will impact the future of the healthcare system.

The Challenge of the Individual Mandate

The Affordable Care Act was passed on March 23, 2010, in President Obama's first term of office. At over 2,500 pages, it was a complex piece of legislation that no one voting for it had completely read. Then House Majority Leader Nancy Pelosi famously pleaded "*We have to pass the bill so we can find out what's in it.*" (March 9, 2010)

One thing that everyone knew was in it was a mandate to force people to purchase health insurance. This "Individual Mandate" was the first time the federal government had ever tried to force Americans to purchase any product in order to be compliant with the law. The Obama administration argued this was in compliance with the so-called Commerce Clause of the Constitution, which gives Congress the power to regulate commerce. But nowhere in the Constitution does it say the government has the authority to *force commerce* upon the American people.

The Individual Mandate was necessary, the White House argued, so that everyone would have health insurance. The truth was that the cost of insurance to cover those with pre-existing medical conditions had to be subsidized by forcing healthy Americans without insurance to buy it. Many of these young people would be coerced into purchasing a product they had never before felt they needed.

To make matters worse, they would have to pay as much as *five times* the actual cost of providing that insurance. This was necessary due to a provision in the law that called for "community rating." That means instead of insurance companies determining their premiums by actuarial analysis (mathematical calculation of the real cost of the insurance), they had to charge the same price to everyone. The only adjustments permitted were for age, tobacco usage, and geographical residence.

Instead of six different premium levels to account for different costs, the insurance companies were forced to come up with only three levels. That meant elderly, sicker patients could not be charged the real cost of their insurance. To compensate, young and healthy patients would have to pay much more. The Obama administration knew this would not encourage participation so they wrote the law to force everyone to purchase insurance.

Republicans saw this portion of the law for what it was; a violation of the Constitution. They insisted you could not compel people to purchase a product and argued this was in reality a tax on the people. A tax would have violated President Obama's promise not to raise taxes on middle and low income Americans. Obama insisted it was not a tax but a fine for failure to comply with the law. He refused to acknowledge he was raising taxes with this new healthcare law.

The issue was challenged in the courts for two years before the Supreme Court finally decided it. The decision surprised both parties.

The Supreme Court Decision

On June 28, 2012, in a 5 to 4 decision, the Court ruled in *NFIB v. Sebelius* that the law was constitutional insofar as the Individual Mandate was concerned; but not because they agreed that Congress could compel individuals to purchase a product.

Chief Justice John Roberts, a conservative, sided with the four liberal justices to form the majority opinion. However, he did not agree with the reasoning of the government that they had the authority to impose a mandate to purchase insurance thus denying their argument this is embodied in the Commerce Clause. Instead, he concluded they were in fact imposing a tax, as Republicans had argued, and the Constitution *did* give them the authority to impose taxes.

Justice Roberts wrote, *"Because the Constitution permits such a tax, it is not our role to forbid it, or to pass upon its wisdom or fairness. Simply put, congress may tax and spend. The federal government may enact a tax on an activity that it cannot authorize, forbid or otherwise control."*

The four other conservative justices had strong dissents. Justices Anthony Kennedy, Samuel Alito, Clarence Thomas, and Antonin Scalia opposed the decision. In his dissent, Kennedy wrote: *"In our view, the entire act before us is invalid in its entirety."* He believed the majority opinion constituted a rewriting of the law. He said, *"What*

Congress calls a penalty, we call a tax. In short, the court imposes a tax when Congress deliberately rejected a tax."

The minority opinion went on to say, *"judicial tax-writing is particularly troubling. . . Taxes have never been popular. . . and in part for that reason, the constitution requires tax increases to originate in the House of Representatives. That is to say, they must originate in the legislative body most accountable to the people, where legislators must weigh the need for the tax against the terrible price they might pay at their next election, which is never more than two years off. . . In a few cases, this court has held that a 'tax' imposed upon private conduct was so onerous as to be in effect a penalty. But we have never held – never - that a penalty imposed for violation of the law was so trivial as to be in effect a tax. We have never held that any exaction imposed for violation of the law is an exercise of Congress's taxing power – even when the statute calls it a tax, much less when (as here) the statute repeatedly calls it a penalty."*

In response to the Supreme Court ruling, former Assistant United States Attorney Andrew C. McCarthy stated:

"Chief Justice Roberts claims that Congress simply used the wrong label. That is legerdemain. This is not a case in which Congress was confused, or inadvertently used the wrong term under circumstances where the error wasn't called to its attention. The tax-or-penalty question was a hotly contested issue. As the dissent points out, it is one thing for a court to construe as a tax an exaction that "bore an agnostic label that does not entail the significant constitutional consequences of a penalty – such as 'license'. . . But we have never – never – treated as a tax an exaction which faces up to the critical difference between a tax and a penalty, and explicitly denominates the exaction a 'penalty'".

He went on to say, *"But today, the Supreme Court rewrote a law – which it has no constitutional authority to do – and treated it as if it were forthrightly, legitimately enacted. Further, it shielded the political branches from accountability for raising taxes, knowing full well that, had Obama and the Democrats leveled with the public that ObamaCare entailed a huge tax hike, it would never have had the votes to pass."*

This ruling upheld the Individual Mandate and the White House celebrated. But lost in the celebration was another important decision in the ruling by the High Court. They also ruled that government did not have the authority to compel the states to expand Medicaid under threat of loss of government subsidies.

The primary purpose of the new healthcare law was to expand the health insurance coverage of all Americans. A large part of that purpose was to be accomplished through the expansion of Medicaid; the government provided health insurance for low-income Americans. This insurance is a cooperative venture between the federal government and the states. The federal government provides varying amounts of support, depending on the financial stability of the states, which averages 57% of the cost of providing health care. The Affordable Care Act (ACA) was written to lower the eligibility standards so as to increase the number of low-income Americans enrolled in the program.

However, in another government over-reach, the Obama administration tried to tie cooperation with the states to government subsidies, threatening to eliminate subsidies to all those states that failed to comply with expansion of Medicaid. The Supreme Court decision struck down this provision of the law and protected state sovereignty. The states would be allowed to make their own decision about Medicaid expansion without fear of loss of federal support.

Why would any state refuse to expand Medicaid eligibility to as many of their residents as possible? The cost of providing Medicaid is one of the largest expenses that every state must reconcile. Unlike the federal government, every state must balance its budget. There is no ability to print money or borrow from other countries to pay the bills.

Even though the ACA provided 100% of the additional cost of Medicaid for the first three years, there was no assurance of federal support in the future. With a federal debt nearing $18 Trillion, many states worried the federal government would be unable to continue their support of Medicaid. That would leave the states with rising Medicaid costs they could not pay. As a result, half of the states elected to forgo expansion of Medicaid.

So this first ruling of the Supreme Court preserved the Individual Mandate, but struck down the threat to the states if they didn't expand Medicaid. These two decisions would have far-reaching implications for the future of ObamaCare.

The Contraception Mandate

The Contraception Mandate refers to the requirements of ObamaCare for all insurance policies to provide contraceptives, sterilization procedures, and abortifacients (drugs that induce abortion). This is part of the "essential health benefits" dictated by the law and determined at the discretion of the HHS Secretary.

After passage of the law in 2010, HHS Secretary Kathleen Sebelius determined that all policies considered compliant with the law would include these controversial benefits. Despite the fact that such drugs are low cost, as little as $9/month and widely available at no cost in many clinics, she insisted every insurance policy sold under ObamaCare must include these benefits.

The response from the Catholic Church was swift and vocal. These benefits violated their religious beliefs and therefore they were unacceptable. After consideration, the White House exempted all churches from the requirements of the law but did not exempt other religious institutions and those individuals and businesses that also objected.

This compromise satisfied no one. Churches were now exempt but the schools they ran were not. Perhaps the most egregious example was the plight of nuns in Colorado. The Little Sisters of the Poor, a Catholic ministry of nuns to the elderly and disabled, was threatened with massive fines if they failed to comply. The fines would be $100/employee/day. This could put them, and others like them, out of business.

Lawsuits Abound

A compromise was again offered, called the "accommodation". This time these institutions would be exempt if they signed documents calling for their insurance company to pick up the tab. This "slight of hand" did nothing to solve the moral dilemma created by this law and this "accommodation" also fell flat. Over one hundred lawsuits were filed on behalf of those affected by this ruling.

The lawsuits fell into two categories: *For-profit* and *Non-profit* businesses and institutions.

For-profit businesses

The *For-profit* lawsuits receiving the most attention included Hobby Lobby, a national chain of arts and crafts stores, and Conestoga Wood Specialties, a cabinet-making company in Pennsylvania.

Both companies are operated by owners with strong religious beliefs that include moral objections to abortifacients. Hobby Lobby is owned by David Green, the son of a pastor from Emporia, Kansas. In 1970 he began making frames for artwork on his kitchen table after noticing customers at the TG&Y store where he worked made paintings on tiny canvases. He put his family to work assembling frames and then opened a retail store two years later.

In 1985 he almost went bankrupt when lenders threatened foreclosure. Green says he crawled under his oak desk and prayed for a way out. Apparently God answered that prayer because today Hobby Lobby has 560 stores and offers up to 90,000 arts, crafts, and home-decor items. Most are not religious but he does stock crosses in a variety of designs and offers Bible school cutouts, and an "armor of God" costume.

The store generates $3.3 Billion in annual sales. The five Green family members that control the company put more than one-third of its profits into religious and other philanthropy according to Mr. Green. The company provides spiritual services for workers and has three chaplains on duty at the company headquarters to pray with workers, provide marriage counseling and recommend the best in newly released Christian films.

The Greens do not object to providing contraceptives to employees but they draw the line when it comes to abortifacients (drugs that induce abortion) and intra-uterine devices that prevent implantation of a fertilized egg. These drugs and devices terminate life after conception and therefore violate the Green's religious convictions.

"I have deeply held convictions, and I should not have to be required by the government to violate my conscience." - David Green, owner of Hobby Lobby.

Conestoga Wood Specialties is owned by Norman and Elizabeth Hahn and their three sons, a Mennonite Christian family from Pennsylvania. According to the web site of their attorneys, Alliance Defending Freedom, the Hahns, *"desire to run the company, a wholesale manufacturer of custom wood kitchen cabinet parts, in a manner that reflects their sincerely held religious beliefs, including their belief that God requires respect for the sanctity of human life."*

Their lawsuits charge that the mandate infringes upon these beliefs and violates their rights as guaranteed by the First Amendment of the Constitution and the Religious Freedom Restoration Act (RFRA) of 1993 by forcing them to pay for employee health insurance that covers such drugs. The RFRA was passed by a voice vote in the House and 97 to 3 in the Senate, and then signed into law by Democratic President Bill Clinton.

The fines for non-compliance with the law are substantial. The penalties are $100/employee/day. For large businesses like Hobby Lobby this amounts to a penalty of $36,000/employee/year or $468 million ($1.3 million/day) for their 13,000 employees. For the Little Sisters of the Poor their fine would be $2.5 million - more than one third of their total annual budget for caring for the sick and elderly.

Many on the left have tried to frame this debate as an attempt to deny women contraceptives. Nothing could be further from the truth. Writing in The American Spectator, David Catron explains:

"These suits have nothing to do with the proposition that corporations are people. Nor do they concern any attempt to force religion on employees or deny women basic contraception coverage. This litigation is about something much larger: whether the government can issue an arbitrary bureaucratic decree that negates a fundamental constitutional right as well as an act of Congress. And no matter how many phony "accommodations" the White House might make, that is the upshot of the contraception mandate. It explains why the legal backlash over the issue has far exceeded that which ObamaCare's individual insurance mandate produced."

These two lawsuits were combined when appealed to the Supreme Court and heard as *Hobby Lobby v. Sebelius* on March 25, 2014. At the time of the writing of my first book on the subject, *The ObamaCare Train Wreck,* the decision of the court was unknown. Now we can discuss their findings.

Supreme Court Upholds Hobby Lobby

On June 30th, 2014, the last day of the session, the Supreme Court of the United States announced its decision in the closely watched Hobby Lobby case. The original case name of *Sebelius v. Hobby Lobby* was changed to *Burwell v. Hobby Lobby* with the new appointment of Sylvia Mathews Burwell as the Secretary of Health and Human Services (HHS). By a 5-4 vote, the Supreme Court ruled in favor of Hobby Lobby, determining that the Affordable Care Act's Contraception Mandate violated their rights under the Religious Freedom Restoration Act (RFRA).

This is a huge victory for Hobby Lobby, Conestoga Wood Specialties, and Mardel Christian Bookstores (also covered in the same lawsuit), but it is an even greater victory for all Americans who value their religious freedom. Unfortunately, many on the left who fought this decision are trying to demonize the supporters of *Hobby Lobby* by distorting the facts of the case. Therefore, it is imperative that we review just what the court decided and what they did not decide.

First, the court did not declare this decision on the basis of the U.S. Constitution. This decision was based on the RFRA. This law stipulates that *"Government may substantially burden a person's exercise of religion **only** if it demonstrates that application of the burden to the person . . . **is the least restrictive means of furthering a compelling governmental interest."***

John Daniel Davidson, writing in *National Review Online* explains the purpose of the RFRA:

*"The purpose of the RFRA was to create a statutory right where a constitutional right doesn't exist – or, at least, is no longer held to exist. The Court's 1990 ruling in **Employment Division v. Smith** upended 30 years of precedent and returned the Court to a standard it first applied in **Reynolds v. United States,** in 1878. In that case, the Court found that a Mormon polygamist in the Utah Territory could not claim that his first Amendment right to free exercise of religion justified his violation of a federal anti-polygamy law. The Court's reasoning, in **Reynolds** and later in **Smith**, was that a generally applicable criminal law does not raise any free-exercise issues whatsoever. That is, the Constitution's free-exercise clause protects religious beliefs but not necessarily religiously motivated actions that run afoul of neutrally enforced federal laws, even if such laws indirectly impeded the exercise of religion."*

In other words, you can't claim a religious freedom from one law in order to break an already established law. For example, if your religion calls for human sacrifices you can't claim that freedom because murder is already an established violation of law that does not target any particular religion.

But the *Smith* decision provoked outrage in Congress and therefore RFRA was passed to re-establish a basis for preserving religious freedom *"unless there was a compelling state interest"*. RFRA says that the burden of proof is on the government to show that the *"compelling state interest"* is served by a law that imposes a significant burden on an individual's religious conduct.

This Supreme Court decision applies to closely-held corporations, essentially family owned businesses, and does not necessarily apply to publically held corporations with numerous stockholders. The Court considers these closely-held corporations as "individuals" and rejects the liberal notion that corporations like these cannot claim religious purposes for their businesses. Justice Samuel Alito, writing for the majority opinion said, "*Protecting the free-exercise rights of corporations like Hobby Lobby, Conestoga, and Mardel protects the religious liberty of the humans who own and control those companies.*"

Liberal Hysteria

Liberals were quick to label this verdict "gender bigotry" as they continue to promote the mythical "war on women." They insist on mischaracterization of the *Hobby Lobby* case and its meaning. John McCormack, writing in *The Weekly Standard* called attention to this hysteria. He writes *Salon* claimed the Court sanctioned "*bosses' denying women all contraception coverage.*" NARAL board member Jessica Valenti declared that the case is "*really about a fear of women's sexuality.*" Steve Coll suggests in *The New Yorker* that the Supreme Court might grant religious exemptions to the Taliban if it organized as a closely-held American corporation.

Even likely presidential candidate Hillary Clinton added to the rhetorical distortions of the Court's decision. McCormack writes, "*At the Aspen Ideas Festival, Clinton warned that the Court had 'introduced this element' into American society usually found in 'very unstable, antidemocratic' countries where men control women's bodies. She lamented that a 'sales clerk at Hobby Lobby who needs contraception, which is pretty expensive, is not going to get that service through her employer's health care.' And, she asked, "Does the decision mean if you're in need of a blood transfusion your insurance policy doesn't have to cover it? This is a really bad slippery slope.*"

So many distortions, where to begin?

First of all, Hobby Lobby provides 16 of 20 FDA-approved contraceptives for all of their employees. They only objected to those 4 contraceptives that destroy a fertilized egg and are therefore considered abortifacients – drugs or devices that induce abortion. Furthermore, the ruling does not prohibit any of their employees from obtaining these abortifacients; it simply exempts the owners from paying for them.

Jonah Goldberg writes in *National Review Online* that abortion-rights protestors gathered outside the Supreme Court building on the day the Court handed down the decisions for *Hobby Lobby* holding signs that read "Birth Control: Not My Boss's Business". But that's precisely the point; it is *not* their bosses' business and the Supreme Court agreed. If you want to take birth control, or even end the conception of a fertilized egg with an abortifacient; that's your business. But don't expect your employer who has religious convictions to the contrary to pay for the choices you make. As Goldberg says, *"The notion that denying a subsidy for a product is equivalent to banning that product is one of the odder tenets of contemporary liberalism."*

As for the expense, contrary to Clinton's statement, the cost of these is approximately $9 per month. McCormack gives perspective on this nominal expense when he says, *"The federal government, which intends to spend $2 Trillion on ObamaCare over the next decade, could scrounge up the change to pay directly for contraceptives or abortifacients not covered by conscientious objectors' health plans."*

What about those blood transfusions Clinton is worried about, or even vaccinations? Justice Alito's majority opinion goes on to say the government could point to *"no evidence that insurance plans in existence prior to the enactment of ACA excluded coverage for such items. Nor has HHS provided evidence that any significant number of employers sought exemption, on religious grounds, from any of ACA's coverage requirements other than the contraceptive mandate."*

The Real Issue

The extreme reactions on the left reveal the true nature of this controversy. It is less about contraceptives and more about abortion. The requirements of the ACA regulations to provide these contraceptives and abortifacients were never passed by Congress. The Obama administration was never able to get the ACA to pay for abortions because several pro-life Democrats refused to vote for that. But the White House tried to get the camel's nose under the tent with the addition of this contraception mandate, which included abortifacients, *after the law was passed.*

These requirements were added under the discretion granted to HHS Secretary Kathleen Sebelius to determine the "*essential health benefits*" the law would require. This particular mandate was developed in conjunction with Planned Parenthood, the largest provider of abortion services in the country. Perhaps this further explains the recent listing of a "dirty 100" organizations by The National Organization of Women (NOW) simply because these companies have filed lawsuits to exempt them from providing these offensive abortifacients. Included in this listing of "dirty" organizations is The Little Sisters of the Poor, nuns who provide desperately needed medical care and comfort to the elderly and disabled. Apparently, NOW doesn't represent *these* women.

Impact on Non-profit Cases

This is a tremendous victory for the *For-profit* companies seeking exemption from the onerous provisions of the ACA. But what about the impact this Court's decision will have on the one hundred *Non-profit* cases pending before the courts? These include The Little Sisters of the Poor, Wheaton College, and Tyndale publishers, just to name a few. Will the Hobby Lobby decision benefit their cases?

The government is actually referencing the *Hobby Lobby* decision in their arguments involving the Wheaton College case. Jess Bravin, writing in *The Wall Street Journal,* says U.S. Solicitor General Donald Verrilli cited the *Hobby Lobby* ruling to buttress the claim it has offered religious non-profits an acceptable compromise to opt out of contraceptive coverage in employee health plans. He is referencing the so-called "accommodation" that was offered by the White House after they received an avalanche of complaints, especially from the Catholic Church, when the requirements of the Contraception Mandate were first released.

But this "accommodation" has been rejected, as it should be, by numerous Christian organizations, as ineffective in relieving the moral objections the law creates. Wheaton responded, *"Wheaton believes that authorizing its (insurance administrator) to provide these drugs in Wheaton's place makes it complicit in grave moral evil. Wheaton can neither provide the mandated coverage nor execute and deliver forms that prompt others to do so."*

Perhaps the most important reaction to the *Hobby Lobby* decision came in a ruling in the Eleventh Circuit Court of Appeals just the day after the Supreme Court decision was handed down. The court was considering the case of Eternal Word Television Network, which runs Catholic-themed programming. *Eternal Word Television Network v. Secretary of HHS* was heard by two left-leaning judges, Beverly Martin and Adalberto Jordan, both appointed by President Bill Clinton, as well as Judge William H. Pryor. The court decided unanimously to grant EWTN its injunctive relief from the burden of the ACA mandate.

Quin Hillyer, writing in *National Review Online,* gives his assessment of the verdict: *"It does not take much to read between the lines in the injunction that a unanimous three-judge panel of the Eleventh Circuit granted Monday afternoon in favor of Eternal Word Television Network. . . . The order begins as follows:* **"In light of the Supreme Court's decision today in the Hobby Lobby case** (emphasis added)*, we grant the motion of Eternal Word Television Network."* Hillyer believes this shows only a grudging acceptance of Monday's undeniable signal from the Supreme Court.

As encouraging as the reaction of these two liberal judges in the EWTN case is, the opinion written by the third judge, William H. Pryor, is even more important. Judge Pryor's 27-page explanation of the verdict covers every possible future argument that might be brought against EWTN in any future court. This is critical for the sake not only of EWTN, but for all *non-profit* religious organizations that seek exemption from the ACA mandate.

Hillyer believes there are three reasons these lawsuits will be favored in future court decisions.

- **One** – The five Supreme Court justices that favored Hobby Lobby will almost certainly favor any future *Non-profit* case deliberations brought to that court.

- **Two** – It is more likely at least two of the four liberal justices of the Supreme Court will join the majority opinion. Actually, all four liberals already joined a unanimous opinion in favor of a church-affiliated school in the *Hosanna-Tabor* case even when the opponent was claiming employment discrimination – a much stronger legal claim than the supposed right to have somebody else subsidize one's contraceptives. Furthermore, two of the four justices refused to join a key part of Justice Ruth Bader Ginsburg's dissent in *Hobby Lobby*.

- **Three** – Judge Pryor's opinion in support of the injunction in *EWTN* is such a tour de force that it provides a perfect template for an eventual Supreme Court decision in favor of the Catholic TV network, leaving no reasonable loopholes to worry the legal conscience of any doubting justices (Anthony Kennedy) on the high court.

Pryor referenced *Hobby Lobby* saying, "*it is not for us to say that (the network's) religious beliefs are mistaken or insubstantial. . . . Courts must instead determine whether the line drawn (by the network) reflects an honest conviction, and there is no dispute that it does.*" Pryor added that the honest conviction of EWTN is that even the so-called "accommodation" offered by HHS will require EWTN's complicity in a scheme that is "*condemned by the principle of material cooperation in evil.*"

Pryor also referenced Pope John Paul II who was approached by the churches in Germany when they were asked to sign "certificates" attesting that women seeking an abortion had first secured "counseling" from the church. In effect, the certificate was used as a prerequisite for an abortion – which is very closely analogous to the "Form 700" that HHS wants EWTN to provide to the insurance provider "in order" for the insurer to provide the abortifacient coverage to which EWTN objects. The Pope ordered the German churches not to comply.

It is clear that Pryor regards the "accommodation" as an ineffective remedy. He writes:

"It is undeniable that the United States has compelled the network to participate in the mandate scheme by requiring the network not only to sign but also to deliver the form to its third-party administrator of its health-insurance plan. The network must sign a form that, on its face, states that the network's delivery of it is required "in order for the plan to be accommodated with respect to the contraceptive coverage requirement."

If the network, or Wheaton College, or The Little Sisters of the Poor, believes that this activity would make them complicit in grave moral sin, who are the courts to adjudicate their own religious convictions?

There is great cause for celebration of the *Hobby Lobby* victory by all Americans who value their religious freedom. But there is also great concern for the future as long as secular progressives like President Obama and his supporters believe the government should be in control of our lives rather than our consciences.

The next important date on the judicial calendar is December 8, 2014, when the U.S. Tenth Circuit Court of Appeals in Denver will hear oral arguments on *Little Sisters of the Poor v. Burwell*. A decision is not expected until June 2015.

The Next Big Threat to ObamaCare

On the same day of March 25, 2014, in the same city where the Supreme Court heard arguments in *Hobby Lobby v. Burwell*, another court was listening to a case that could have far more significant impact on the future of ObamaCare. In the 10th Circuit Court of Appeals in Washington, D. C., lawyers for both sides in the case known as *Halbig v. Burwell* presented their arguments.

The case is all about eligibility for subsidies for those individuals purchasing health insurance on the government exchanges. The law was written to stipulate that those who would receive subsidies must do so on state-run exchanges. Those who signed up on federal exchanges would not be eligible for subsidies. This was not an unintended consequence.

When ObamaCare was debated in the Congress, there was much disagreement on this issue. *The Wall Street Journal* editorial board clarified this issue in the days just prior to the court's hearing of the case in March. They wrote:

"The Affordable Care Act – at least the version that passed in 2010 – instructed the states to establish insurance exchanges, and if they didn't the Health and Human Services Department was authorized to build federal exchanges. The law says that subsidies will be available only to people who enroll "through an Exchange established by the State." The question in Halbig is whether these taxpayer subsidies can be distributed through the federal exchanges, as the Administration insists."

They explain that Democrats were divided over the structure of the exchanges, with liberals favoring federal exchanges and moderates favoring state control. Senator Ben Nelson (D-NE) held the key vote and was concerned about excessive federal control of the exchanges. The federalists (those upholding states' rights) won and conditioned the subsidies on state-based exchanges. The Constitution preserves the rights of states to their own sovereignty so Democrats created an incentive for Governors to participate voluntarily.

They established a *quid pro quo* to encourage participation. If they didn't cooperate by establishing state exchanges, they wouldn't be eligible for the billion of dollars of subsidies for their constituents. The administration also hoped the states would pick up much of the work of implementing the exchanges rather than forcing HHS to do the work instead. The White House was so convinced of the merits of the law they never dreamed the states would object to this provision.

But they were sadly mistaken. Rather than submit to this *quid pro quo*, 34 states opted out. At present, only 16 states and the District of Columbia established their own exchanges. Many of these have since failed. (See Chapter One) This left the White House with a dilemma; obey the law denying subsidies to approximately two-thirds of the population and consequently threaten the survival of the system; or ignore the law and provide subsidies to those signing up on the federal exchanges. They ignored the law, arguing Congress actually intended the subsidies to be available to all. This argument holds little water when you recognize that the restrictive language appears no less than nine times in the text of the law.

Recent Court Rulings

The plaintiffs in *Halbig v. Burwell* are individuals and small businesses in six states that didn't establish state exchanges. They objected to the White House's rewriting of the law because, without the subsidies, the plaintiffs could have claimed exemptions from the Individual Mandate tax. That's because the law exempts those individuals whose cost of obtaining insurance exceeds 8% of their income. But with these subsidies, many of these individuals and small businesses are no longer exempt.

Recent court rulings give encouragement to their cause. In a recent Op-Ed for *The Los Angeles Times,* liberal constitutional law professor Jonathan Turley cites important evidence of the Supreme Court's sympathies:

*"In **Michigan v. Bay Mills Indian Community**, for example, Justice Elena Kagan noted that "this court does not revise legislation . . . just because the text as written creates an apparent anomaly as to some subject it does not address." In **Utility Air Regulatory Group v. EPA**, Justice Antonin Scalia, writing for the majority, stressed that "an agency has no power to tailor legislation to bureaucratic policy goals by rewriting unambiguous*

*statutory terms." And a third strike came last week in **National Labor Relations Board v. Canning**, when the Supreme Court unanimously found that President Obama had violated the Constitution in circumventing Congress through his use of recess appointments."*

Turley, an Obama supporter, has nevertheless been critical of the president's overreach on executive powers.

Others agreed with Turley's assessment. Jeffrey Dorfman, writing for *Forbes,* cited these same recent rulings and believes ObamaCare is facing a major setback and even a possible collapse. He sums up the situation as follows:

*"While everyone focuses on the impact of **Utility Air Regulatory Group v. EPA** on the government's power to address climate change, the Supreme Court may have done more to impact the future of ObamaCare with their ruling than they did to impact the future of the world's climate."*

The Impact of a *Halbig* Victory

Turley believes the impact of a *Halbig* victory is hard to overstate. Without subsidies, those individuals in the 34 states without exchanges would face huge additional costs and many would drop their health insurance. Many of these, like the *Halbig* plaintiffs, would then be eligible for exemptions from the Individual Mandate. All of this would raise the cost of health insurance for all those purchasing coverage. This would reawaken fears in the insurance industry of the "death spiral" when not enough people purchase insurance to defray the costs of their medical expenses.

Rising insurance costs would increase the need for government bailouts of the insurance industry even more than has already happened. The public's reaction to this situation would surely provoke a Congressional overhaul and possible repeal of ObamaCare.

John Fund, writing for *National Review Online*, believes some states would move to set up their own exchanges, perhaps benefiting from the lessons of ObamaCare's shaky rollout. But he also states the Obama administration would have no choice but to work with Congress as it revisited the exchange issue and rewrote the law. He concludes:

*"A favorable ruling in **Halbig** by the Supreme Court might be just the two-by-four needed to get President Obama's attention and make him realize that his pen has run out of enforcement ink."*

White House Desperation

You might wonder why the Obama administration would risk such an adverse ruling in the courts. Why try to get by with such an obvious re-interpretation of the plain language of the law?

Since the law exempts people from the Individual Mandate tax whose cost of insurance exceeds 8% of their income, many of these people would have chosen not to purchase insurance. This possibility posed an existential threat to the future of ObamaCare.

Even more threatening to the Obama White House was the possibility this could jeopardize the President's re-election campaign in 2012. Therefore the White House looked to the IRS to solve their problem.

According to Kimberley A. Strassel, writing in *The Wall Street Journal,* in the late summer of 2010 after passage of ObamaCare, the IRS assembled a working group whose initial intent was to follow the text of the law. An early draft of its rule about subsidies explained that they were for "Exchanges established by the State."

But in March 2011, when it became evident that 36 states were not establishing their own exchanges, everything changed. IRS officials began focusing on a new interpretation of the health care law. The office of the IRS chief counsel, a political appointee, drafted a memo telling the group that the text should be interpreted to mean that everyone, in every exchange, got subsidies. Some time between March 10 and March 15, 2011, the reference to "Exchanges established by the State" disappeared from the draft rule.

Clearly concerned about the legality of this new interpretation, the IRS sought coverage for its predetermined political goal. A March 27,

2011 email has IRS employees asking HHS political hires to cover the tax agency's backside by issuing its own rule deeming HHS-run exchanges to be state-run exchanges. HHS complied with their request in July 2011. One month later the IRS put out its ruling that provided subsidies for all.

Strassel summarizes this illegal activity thus:

"The IRS (famed for nitpicking and prosecuting the tax law), chose to authorize hundreds of billions of illegal subsidies without having performed a smidgen of legal due diligence, and did so at the direction of political taskmasters. The agency's actions provided aid and comfort to elected Democrats, even as it disenfranchised millions of Americans who voted in their states to reject state-run exchanges. And Treasury knows how ugly this looks, which is why it initially stonewalled Congress in its investigation – at first refusing to give documents to investigators, and redacting large portions of the information."

Law professor Jonathan Adler of Case Western Reserve and Michael Cannon of the Cato Institute first called attention to this IRS abuse in an Op-Ed article in *The Wall Street Journal* in 2011. In a follow-up article recently, they write, *"At its heart, though, Halbig is not just about ObamaCare. It is about determining whether the president, like an autocrat, can levy taxes on his own authority."*

The White House strategy to defend this lawlessness is to claim it was the original intent of Congress to provide subsidies to everyone. Therefore they are merely implementing the law as Congress intended. In their defense, the liberal 4th Circuit Court applied this interpretation to the law in upholding the government's position in *King v. Burwell*.

However, this is clearly a fabrication of the truth. Recently **video evidence** was found that gives insider testimony indicating Congress never intended for subsidies to be received on the federal exchanges. Jonathan Gruber, MIT economist and one of the authors of ObamaCare, made at least two public appearances after the law was passed by Congress in which he said:

"If you're a state and you don't set up an exchange, that means your citizens don't get their tax credits. I hope that that's a blatant enough political reality that states will get their act together and realize there are billions of dollars at stake here in setting up these exchanges."

As you might expect, Gruber is now trying to walk back those remarks much like Hillary Clinton is now trying to distance herself from the foreign policy of President Obama. But if we're to believe that they weren't telling the truth before, why should we believe they're telling the truth now?

Court Upholds the Law

On July 22nd, the D. C. Circuit Court of Appeals upheld the law as written and found in favor of *Halbig*.

The White House had argued that the law was ambiguous. But *The Wall Street Journal* editorial staff makes it clear there is no ambiguity in the law as written. The majority opinion agreed.

Judge Thomas Griffith, speaking for the majority in the *Halbig v. Burwell* decision, admitted they reached their decision *"frankly, with reluctance"* considering the consequences. *"But, high as those stakes are, the principle of legislative supremacy that guides us is higher still. Within constitutional limits, Congress is supreme in matters of policy, and the consequence of that supremacy is that our duty when interpreting a statute is to ascertain the meaning of the words of the statute duly enacted through the formal legislative process."*

White House Moves to Delay

The Obama administration moved to delay any further judicial action that might impact ObamaCare. The Solicitor General, Donald B. Verrilli, Jr., asked the D. C. Circuit Court to vacate its own decision in *Halbig v. Burwell* by accepting a request for an *en banc* review.

The D. C. Circuit Court struck down the Obama administration interpretation of the law in its decision of *Halbig v. Burwell* when two of three justices on the panel found the law to be clear and the Obama administration violated the law. In response, the White House called for an *en banc* review, which means not just three justices but the whole court of eleven will hear the case. Democrats have been anticipating such a situation for a long time and Senate Majority Leader Harry Reid was ready.

Senator Reid's Agenda

This played into the hand of Senator Reid, who stacked the D. C. Circuit Court for just such a situation, when he called for the "nuclear option" by striking down the Senate filibuster rule that had existed since 1837. Though both parties had decried this rule when their majority position was stymied by the minority party, both recognized the importance of it in assuring the rights of the minority. Reid, himself, had argued vociferously when his party was in the minority that the rule was important to maintain.

But on November 21, 2013, Reid destroyed nearly 200 years of Senate precedent and ended the filibuster rule for appointment of judges at all levels except the Supreme Court. His reason for doing it was precisely to set up the situation we find now in the D. C. Circuit Court. By railroading through 3 liberal judges on a party-line vote that could not be achieved with the filibuster rule, he has packed the Court with a liberal majority of seven to four. True to their liberal ideology, the court struck down the initial decision of the three-judge panel and accepted the case for *en banc* review, even though this occurs only once in every 500 cases.

The *en banc* review was actually scheduled to take place the week before Christmas, 2014 which further satisfied the Obama administration desire to delay the impact. The IRS is currently granting subsidies to millions of Americans unlawfully and will continue to do so as the slow judicial process plays out. The White House was hoping the longer they delayed the more likely the Court will find in their favor.

King v. Burwell

However, another judicial review was playing out on a parallel course on the same issue. *King v. Burwell* was decided in the 4th Circuit

Court in Virginia and the government won this decision. The Court reluctantly found in favor of the government when they interpreted the "intention of Congress" as the White House argued.

But ironically, this victory by the White House gave momentum to an appeal to the Supreme Court for the ultimate arbitration of the issue. *The Wall Street Journal* reports Michael Carvin, the lead attorney in both *King* and *Halbig,* filed a cert petition asking the Supreme Court to hear *King.* Carvin reasoned that if the Supreme Court will hear the issue this term then the *en bank* review of *Halbig* will be rendered irrelevant.

"There is no value to further percolation," says Joshua Hawley and several other former clerks for Chief Justice John Roberts in a well-argued amicus brief for the *King* cert petition. The Journal editorial board said, *"The legal questions are uncomplicated and squarely in front of the Supreme Court. But the legal uncertainty is bleeding into health markets already, and if the illegal subsidies are ultimately withdrawn, the disruptions to individuals and businesses will be that much worse after a legal-political lag of several years. The country would be better off with a quick, decisive resolution. And however the Justices rule, they would send a message to Mr. Reid to stay out of their chambers."*

President Obama, and his enablers like Mr. Reid, have repeatedly shown contempt for the Judiciary and the Constitution with unilateral moves such as this one to circumvent the law as it suits their political agenda. It is hoped that the Supreme Court will again put a stop to such lawlessness and uphold the law as it was written. The Constitution ultimately provides for the means to change laws that need changing – by the votes of the people.

Pruitt v. Burwell

Another judicial decision on the same matter was handed down from the State of Oklahoma. Oklahoma Attorney General Scott Pruitt won a victory in his lawsuit in the Oklahoma U.S. District Court in a ruling that upheld the law as written, again. This decision agrees with the original *Halbig v. Burwell* ruling.

U. S. District Court Judge Ronald White stated, *"The court holds that the IRS rule is arbitrary, capricious, and abuse of discretion or otherwise not in accordance with law . . . . the court is upholding the Act as written. Congress is free to amend the ACA to provide for tax credits in both state and federal exchanges, if that is the legislative will."*

Judge White explains further: *"The alternative leads us down a path toward Alice's Wonderland, where up is down and down is up, and words mean anything."*

The Wall Street Journal editorial board opines that the White House would prefer that ObamaCare remain in such a legal wonderland for as long as possible. But this ruling puts more pressure on the Supreme Court to hear the issue and make a final determination. *"The relevant questions are now squarely in front of the Supreme Court, and for the sake of the law and the future of heath policy the Justices should accept an appeal for the King case for their term that begins next week."*

Chris Conover writes in *Forbes* that the odds are strong that the Supreme Court would uphold the law as written just as Judge White ruled. Even liberal Supreme Court Justice Elena Kagan has previously upheld legislation as written in *Michigan v. Bay Mills Indian Community.* She wrote *"This court does not revise legislation . . . just because the text as written creates an apparent anomaly as to some subject it does not address. . . This Court has no roving license, in even ordinary cases of statutory interpretation, to disregard clear language simply on the view that . . . congress 'must have intended' something broader. . . Congress of course may always change its mind – and we would readily defer to that new decision . . . We will not rewrite Congress's handiwork."*

Justices Scalia and Roberts are also on record with similar views in similar cases. In *Utility Air Regulatory Group v. EPA,* they wrote *"We reaffirm the core administrative-law principle that an agency may not rewrite clear statutory terms to suit its own sense of how the statute should operate."*

The Impact of the Decision

Shortly before this book went to print, the Supreme Court *did* accept *King v. Burwell* for oral arguments in this term of the court. The High Court heard oral arguments on March 4th, 2015. That means a decision will be handed down by the end of the court's term in June 2015.

Michael Cannon, writing in *Forbes,* says the overturning of the IRS interpretation of the law will have monumental repercussions. He estimates this would free over 8 million Americans from the burden of the individual mandate along with 57 million workers from the burden of these mandates. The Congressional Research Service says such a ruling *"could be a major obstacle to the implementation of the Act."*

Such a ruling would necessitate re-writing of the law to comply with the White House's desire to extend these subsidies to everyone on the federal exchanges. But that would require the cooperation of a Republican Congress more interested in repealing the law than changing it to suit President Obama. This opens the door for Republicans to propose major changes to the law even before pushing their repeal agenda, which would require a Republican president in 2017.

Ironically, when the Supreme Court decides the case, Chief Justice John Roberts will get a second bite of the apple to honor his famous words spoken when the court reviewed the Individual Mandate. He said in 2012, *"It is not our job to protect the people from the consequences of their political choices."*

House v. Burwell

The most recent lawsuit concerning ObamaCare is *House v. Burwell,* a case filed by the House of Representatives against the Obama administration that asks a federal court to invalidate two actions by President Obama that it claims violate the Affordable Care Act. This lawsuit, much like *King v. Burwell,* concerns subsidies paid to people purchasing health insurance on the Exchanges.

House claims the president cannot issue "cost-sharing subsidies" in *any* state, because Congress never appropriated funds for those subsidies. Cannon explains that spending federal dollars not pursuant to a congressional appropriation is a federal crime. It would block $3 Billion in subsidies this year, and $175 Billion over the next 10 years. The House also claims the president violated the law by unilaterally delaying the obligations the ACA imposes on employers by delaying the onset of the employer mandate past the date specified in the statute.

Cannon summarizes the impact of the two cases:

*"Thus, both **King** and **House** would block the $2 billion ($126 billion/10 years) in "cost-sharing subsidies" the administration is issuing in the 36 federal-Exchange states. But while **King** would also block the $7 billion ($523billion/10 years) in "premium-assistance tax credits" the administration is issuing in those 36 states, **House** would block the $1 billion ($49 billion/10 years) in "cost-sharing subsidies" the administration is issuing in the 14 states that established Exchanges."*

In simpler language, he says, *"Put differently, **King** would knock out two legs of the ACA's three-legged stool in 36 states. **House** would at least shorten one of those legs in all 50 states."*

It is clear that the judicial system has been busy evaluating the impact and interpretation of ObamaCare – and its work is far from finished. With the recent Republican wave in the mid-term elections (see Chapter Fifteen), the question now is whether this law will be struck down first in the courts or later in the halls of Congress.

Trampling the Constitution

"I was a constitutional law professor, which means unlike the current president, I actually respect the Constitution."
Presidential candidate Barack Obama, 3/30/07

"I do solemnly swear (or affirm) that I will faithfully execute the Office of President of the United States, and will to the best of my ability, preserve, protect and defend the Constitution of the United States."
(Article 2, Section 1, Clause 8)
Presidential Oath of Office,
Sworn by Barack Obama, 1/20/09 and 1/21/13

It is ironic that we have a constitutional lawyer for a president. Despite his campaign rhetoric to the contrary, his actions as president have repeatedly challenged the Constitution, forcing Congress and others to use the Judicial branch of our government to stop him.

There are many critics of Obama's claim to be a constitutional lawyer, from both political parties. The Republican National Committee challenged his claim saying his position at The University of Chicago Law School was "senior lecturer" and not "professor". The Hillary Clinton campaign also challenged this assertion, stating there is a vast difference between the two titles.

FactCheck.org reviewed the matter and found a statement from the U C Law School that defended Obama's characterization of his status. They stated that he had been a "Senior Lecturer" from 1996 to 2004 during which time he taught three courses per year. *"Senior Lecturers are considered to be members of the Law School faculty and are regarded as professors, although not full-time or tenure-track. The title of Senior Lecturer is distinct from the title of Lecturer, which signifies adjunct status. Like Obama, each of the Law School's Senior Lecturers have high-demand careers in politics or public service, which prevent full-time teaching."*

Yet despite this affirmation of his credentials, it is alarming to see how this president has repeatedly shown his disdain for the same foundational document of our government that he taught others, and criticized President Bush, to respect.

Three Branches of Government

Any high school student of civics can tell you we have three branches of government: Executive, Legislative, and Judicial. Laws are made in the Legislative branch and carried out by the Executive branch. When there are differences of opinion on these laws they are settled by the Judicial branch. Laws are not made by the Executive branch.

The Executive branch proposes laws to the Legislative branch, Congress, which are then passed by elected representatives of the people. It is not the role of the Executive branch, the President, to make laws or choose which ones he will or will not enforce. If he does, he destroys the framework of our republic and makes himself out to be a dictator. This issue goes to the core of what makes us a democracy and what separates us from so-called "banana republics" where dictators determine what the laws will be.

Charles Krauthammer, highly respected syndicated columnist for *The Washington Post,* used just such an analogy in an interview on Fox News. In commenting on the latest Obama unilateral change of ObamaCare he said,

"This is stuff you do in a banana republic. It's as if the law is simply a blackboard on which Obama writes any number he wants, any delay he wants on any provision."

Changes to the Affordable Care Act

In *The ObamaCare Train Wreck* I chronicled the changes President Obama made to the Affordable Care Act through February 10, 2014. By that time there were 35 changes to the law, 18 unlawfully made by President Obama, 15 made by Congress, and 2 as a result of decisions of the Supreme Court.

For clarity, I have summarized them again here:

Changes Made by President Obama

These changes were made unilaterally by President Obama without Congressional approval:

1. Medicare Advantage patch – (April 19, 2011)

The original legislation called for cuts of $156 Billion in spending for Medicare Advantage plans. These popular plans for low-income seniors currently account for 28 % of Medicare enrollment. But with these cuts, the Medicare actuary estimates 7.5 Million will lose their plans, or half of the current 15 Million enrolled. To forestall these cuts in benefits and delay the early exit of these plans, the Obama administration ordered an advance draw on funds from a Medicare bonus program to provide extra payment to Medicare Advantage plans, temporarily.

2. Employee reporting – (January 1, 2012)

A one-year delay of the requirement that employers must report to their employees on their W-2 forms the full cost of their employer-provided health insurance, was declared by the Obama Administration.

3. Subsidies may flow through federal exchanges – (May 23, 2012)

The original ObamaCare legislation says the premium assistance tax credits, for those who are eligible, are only available on state run insurance exchanges. They cannot be accessed through federal exchanges. After half the states refused to set up state exchanges, the Obama Administration IRS issued a rule allowing these subsides to be available on federal exchanges.

4. Closing the high-risk pool – (February 15, 2013)

The Obama Administration decided to halt enrollment in transitional federal high-risk pools created by the law, blocking coverage for an estimated 40,000 new applicants, citing a lack of funds. However, the administration had money from a fund under Secretary Sebelius's control but instead used the money to pay for advertising for ObamaCare enrollment. The result will be higher premiums for everyone to cover these high-risk individuals who have to be absorbed in the general insurance population.

5. Doubling allowed deductibles – (February 20, 2013)

Maximum out-of-pocket expenses were capped by the original legislation. But because some group health plans use more than one benefits administrator, plans are now allowed to apply separate patient cost-sharing limits to different services, such as doctor/hospital visits and prescription drugs. The next effect is to double the out-of-pocket expenses for these individuals, which will hurt lower income Americans especially.

6. Small businesses on hold – (March 11, 2013)

The original law called for the establishment of a Small Employer Health Option Program (SHOP) to allow small businesses to purchase insurance at cheaper rates comparable to large businesses. However, the federal government failed to set up the federal exchanges to provide this service so the Obama Administration delayed the requirement for SHOP to offer a choice of qualified health plans until 2015. The result will be small businesses paying more for insurance premiums to cover their employees.

7.Delaying a low-income plan – (March 22, 2013)

The administration delayed implementation of the Basic Health Program until 2015. It would have provided more- affordable health coverage for certain low-income individuals not eligible for Medicaid.

8. *Employer Mandate delayed – (July 2, 2013)*

Over the holiday weekend, the White House released this latest delay in a Treasury Department blog, extending a key provision of the law, the Employer Mandate, by one year. The mandate was set to take effect on January 1, 2014, but was delayed by this unilateral action of President Obama until January 1, 2015, after the November 2014 mid-term elections. The Individual Mandate, however, was not delayed despite pressure from both parties.

9. *Self-attestation – (July 15, 2013)*

Subsidies are available on the exchanges to those individuals who qualify based on their income. To be eligible, you must have an income greater than 133 % of the Federal Poverty Level (FPL) and less than 400 % of FPL. The original law called for income verification by the IRS based on the data provided to them by employers. But after the delay of the reporting requirements of employers (See #2 above) the Obama Administration decided to waive the income verification rules and allow "self-attestation" of income. The likelihood of wide spread fraud caused an outrage from Congress and the public and this change was partially retracted.

10. *Delaying the online SHOP exchange – (November 27, 2013)*

The administration first delayed for a month and later for a year until November 2014, the launch of the online insurance market place for small businesses. The exchange was originally scheduled to launch on October 1, 2013.

11. *Congressional opt-out – (September 30, 2013)*

By the terms of the original law, the members of Congress and the White House staff would be subject to the same insurance on the exchanges and the same subsidies as every other American. But the Obama Administration decided to offer Congressional and White House staff better insurance with higher subsidies on the federal exchanges. They became eligible for subsidies even with incomes up to $174,000/year while everyone else was subject to caps on subsidies at 400 % of FPL or about $94,000 for a family of four.

12. Delaying the Individual Mandate – (October 23, 2013)
The original law called for penalties to be assessed for those individuals who failed to purchase insurance by mid-February, 2014. The administration changed the deadline to March 31, 2014.

13. Insurance companies may offer canceled plans – (November 14, 2013)
After the disastrous roll-out of the law in October, over 6 million Americans found their health insurance had been cancelled. A public outrage ensued so the White House announced that insurance companies may re-offer plans that previous regulations forced them to cancel. No consultation with insurance companies or state insurance commissioners nor Congressional approved was sought.

14. Exempting unions from reinsurance fee – (December 2, 2013)
A reinsurance tax of $63/policyholder was assessed by the original legislation as a means subsidizing any insurance company losses in the early years of the legislation. Unions balked at this disclosure and the Obama Administration, heavily supported by union donations, acceded to their demands. They gave the unions an exemption from this tax. To make up for this exemption, non-exempt plans will have to pay a higher fee, which will likely be passed on to consumers in the form of higher premiums and deductibles. More crony capitalism.

15. Extending Preexisting Condition Insurance Plan – (December 12, 2013) (January 14, 2014)
The administration extended the federal high-risk pool until January 31, 2014, and again until March 15, 2014, to prevent a

coverage gap for the most vulnerable. The plans were scheduled to expire on December 31, but were extended because it has been impossible for some to sign up for new coverage due to the failure of the government web site, healthcare.gov.

16. Expanding catastrophic hardship waiver to those with canceled plans – (December 19, 2013)

The administration expanded the hardship waiver, which allows some people to purchase catastrophic health insurance, to people who have had their plans canceled because of ObamaCare regulations. This is only a temporary fix so these plans will again be illegal in 2015, conveniently after the November 2014 mid-term elections. Compassion or political strategy?

17. Equal employer coverage delayed – (January 18, 2013)

Tax officials will not be enforcing in 2014 the mandate requiring employers to offer equal coverage to all their employees. This provision of the law was supposed to go into effect in 2010, but IRS officials have "yet to issue regulations for employers to follow." It is now nearly four full years since the law was signed by President Obama and the IRS still is incapable of issuing these regulations?

18. Employer Mandate delayed again – (February 10, 2014)

Once again, the Obama Administration had delayed the Employer Mandate, this time until January 1, 2016. They have postponed enforcement of the requirement for medium-sized companies of 50-99 employees and relaxed some additional requirements for larger companies with over 100 employees. Businesses with over 100 employees now only have to offer coverage to 70% of their full-time employees in 2015 and 95 % in 2016 and beyond. There can be no doubt that the specter of millions of employees receiving insurance policy cancellation notices just before the November elections influenced the White House to make this unilateral change.

Changes Made by Congress

These changes were made by Congress and signed by President Obama:

19. Military benefits – (April 26, 2010)

Congress clarified that plans provided by TRICARE, the military's health-insurance program, constitutes minimal essential health-care coverage as required by ObamaCare; its benefits and plans wouldn't normally meet the ACA requirements.

20. VA benefits – (May 27, 2010)

Congress also clarified that health care provided by the Department of Veterans Affairs constitutes minimum essential health-care coverage as required by the ACA.

21. Drug Price clarification – (August 10, 2010)

Congress modified the definition of average manufacturer price (AMP) to include inhalation, infusion, implanted, or injectable drugs that are not generally dispensed through a retail pharmacy.

22. Doc-fix tax – (December 15, 2010)

Congress modified the amount of premium tax credits that individuals would have to repay if they are over-allotted, an action designed to help offset the costs of the postponement of cuts in Medicare physician payments called for in the ACA.

23. Extending the adoption credit – (December 17, 2010)

Congress extended the nonrefundable adoption tax credit, which happened to be included in the ACA, through tax year 2012.

24. TRICARE for adult children – (January 7, 2011)

Congress extended TRICARE coverage to dependent adult children up to age 26 when it had previously only covered those up to the age of 21 - though beneficiaries still have to pay premiums for them.

25. 1099 repealed – (April 14, 2011)

Congress repealed the paperwork ("1099") mandate that would have required businesses to report to the IRS all of their transactions with vendors totaling $600 or more in a year. This would have been a huge additional expense that would especially burden small businesses.

26. No free-choice vouchers – (April 15, 2011)

Congress repealed a program, supported by Senator Ron Wyden (D - Oregon) that would have allowed "free-choice vouchers," that *The Hill* warned "could lead young, healthy workers to opt out" of their employer plans, "driving up costs for everybody else." The same law barred additional funds for the IRS to hire new agents to enforce the health-care law.

27. No Medicaid for well-to-do seniors – (November 21, 2011)

Congress saved taxpayers $13 Billion by changing how the eligibility for certain programs is calculated under ObamaCare. Without the change, a couple earning as much as $64,000 would still have been able to qualify for Medicaid.

28. CO-OPS, IPAB, IRS defunded – (December 23, 2011)

Congress made further cuts to agencies implementing ObamaCare. It trimmed another $400 million off the CO-OP program, cut another $305 million form the IRS to hamper its ability to enforce the law's tax hikes and mandates, and rescinded $10 million in funding for the controversial Independent Payment Advisory Board (IPAB).

29. Slush -fund savings – (February 22, 2012)

Congress slashed another $11.6 Billion from the Prevention and Public Health slush fund and $2.5 Billion from ObamaCare's "Louisiana Purchase," a promise to Louisiana Senator Mary Landrieu made to insure her vote on the original legislation.

30. Less cash for Louisiana – (July 6, 2012)

Congress slashed an additional $670 million from the "Louisiana Purchase" promise made to Senator Mary Landrieu five months later.

31. CLASS Act eliminated – (January 2, 2013)

The original ObamaCare bill called for fund to promote long-term care insurance called the Community Living Assistance Services and Supports (CLASS). The program quickly became unsustainable and even the White House admitted it was fiscally irresponsible. The Democratic chairman of the Senate Finance Committee, Max Baucus, called it "a Ponzi scheme of the first order."

32. Cutting CO-OPS – (January 2, 2013)

Congress cut $2.2 Billion from the "Consumer Operated and Oriented Plan" (CO-OP), which some saw as a stealth public option, blocking creation of government-subsidized co-op insurance programs in about half the states. Early reports showed many co-ops, which had received federal loans, had run into serious financial trouble.

33. Trimming the Medicare trust-fund transfer – (March 26, 2013)

Congress rescinded $200 million of the $500 million scheduled to be taken from the Medicare Part A and Part B trust funds and sent to the Community-Based Care Transition Program established and funded by the ACA.

Changes Made by The Supreme Court
These changes came about with the ruling of The Supreme Court on the constitutionality of ObamaCare: (NFIB v. Sebelius)

34. Medicaid expansion voluntary – (June 28, 2012)

ObamaCare sought to force all states to expand their Medicaid programs with new eligibility rules and planned to punish those states that were non-compliant by withholding funding of current

Medicaid enrollees. The court ruled it had to be voluntary, rather than mandatory, for states to expand Medicaid eligibility to people with incomes up to 133 % of FPL, by ruling that the federal government couldn't halt funds for existing state Medicaid programs if they chose not to participate. The result of this change is about half the states chose not to participate.

35. The Individual Mandate changed to a tax – (June 28, 2012)

The court determined that violating the mandate that Americans must purchase government-approved health insurance would only result in individuals' paying a "tax," making it, legally speaking, optional for people to comply. The Obama Administration had described the consequences of non-compliance as a "penalty," but Chief Justice Roberts ruled it constitutional on the basis that it was actually a tax, not a penalty.

***

More Changes Made by President Obama

These changes occurred after February 10, 2014, and were also made without Congressional approval. They were made after publication of my earlier book, The ObamaCare Train Wreck:

36. Bay State Bailout – (February, 2014)

More than 300,000 people in Massachusetts gained temporary Medicaid coverage in 2014 without any verification of their eligibility, with the Obama and Patrick administrations using a taxpayer-funded bailout to mask the failure of the commonwealth's disastrously malfunctioning website. (more in Chapter One)

37. Extending Subsidies to Non-exchange Plans – (February 27, 2014)

The Obama administration released a bulletin through CMS extending subsidies to individuals who purchased health insurance plans outside of the federal or state exchanges. The bulletin also requires retroactive coverage and subsidies for individuals from the date they applied on the marketplace rather than the date they actually enrolled in a plan. (Chapter Two – *Halbig v. Burwell*)

38. Non-compliant Health Plans Get Two Year Extension – (March 5, 2014)

The Obama administration granted a further delay in enforcement of the law concerning the requirements of the insurance policies. These "illegal" plans may now be offered until 2017.

The Wall Street Journal editorial board called this latest change, *The Endangered Senators Rule,* for its undeniable political motivation. The HHS removed all shadow of a doubt about its motivation when they distributed to reporters a backgrounder noting that the new rule was *"developed in close consultation with members of Congress."* Included in the fact sheet was mention of Senators by name *"including but not limited to"* Mary Landrieu, Mark Udall, Mark Warner, and Jeanne Shaheen, plus nine House Democrats, all running for re-election in the November mid-terms.

They concluded by saying, *"Whether or not this temporary regulatory leniency avoids more insurance disruption the gambit shows the White House is terrified of a Republican Senate that would be rightly viewed as an ObamaCare repudiation. Now it is even willing to pose as an ideological Saint Augustine: ObamaCare cancels all noncompliant plans because letting people keep the plans they like is a threat to government control - just don't cancel them yet."*

39. Reducing Cost-Sharing Deductions – (March 11, 2014)

The ACA originally called for out-of-pocket maximums to be lowered for enrollees with incomes between 100-400% of FPL. (Sec. 1402), but the provision proved unworkable for those 250-400% of FPL in combination with prescribed actuarial value requirements and was changed through regulation to apply to only those 100-250% of poverty.

40. Delaying the Sign-up Deadline – (March 26, 2014)

Allows anyone with virtually any "hardship" to qualify for a waiver past the open enrollment deadline until the hardship can be accommodated. Applicants simply need to check a box on their application to qualify for this extension. This appears to be an open-ended waiver that will undermine the Individual Mandate.

In yet another political move, President Obama further delayed the impact of the Individual Mandate, despite repeated claims by the White House there would be no further delays. Anyone seeking an extension will be granted one on "the honor system" with no need for documentation of the reason for an extension.

The Wall Street Journal editorial board called this for what it is – an opportunity for people to be dishonest:

"All of this is an invitation for people to game the system and wait until they become ill or are injured to sign up for insurance. Much like the rules that destroyed the individual insurance markets in states like New York, Washington and Kentucky, ObamaCare's mandates prevent Americans from being accountable for their own health-care decisions. The new delay ensures that the uncertainty will be built into higher premiums, and insurers must act on incomplete information.

This pattern of dishonesty and political improvisation has come to define ObamaCare, which is the law for some people, sometimes, except when it isn't. Nothing HHS claims can be trusted, and little that the President of the United States promised about his signature law has turned out to be true."

41. Canceling Medicare Advantage Cuts – (April 7, 2014)

In another blatantly political move, President Obama canceled scheduled cuts to the Medicare Advantage plans. The ACA calls for $200 Billion in cuts to Medicare Advantage over 10 years. These popular plans with seniors currently cover about 15 million Americans. The cuts in ObamaCare are expected to cause 7 million seniors to lose their Medicare Advantage plans. This unlawful change by Obama delays this impact until after the November 2014 mid-term elections.

42. More Funds for Insurer Bailout – (May 16, 2014)

The Obama administration said it will supplement risk corridor payments to health insurance plans with "other sources of funding" if the higher risk profile of enrollees means the plans would lose money.

The President does not have the authority to make this change in the law nor to take funds from other sources to pay for it. This is simply another over-reach by the Executive branch into the powers of Congress. The clear reason for this move is to protect insurance company losses to ensure that premiums are not raised to reflect the true cost of the insurance. The American taxpayers will just pick up the tab for the losses.

43. Exempting U.S. Territories – (July 18, 2014)

Despite earlier administration claims that "HHS is not authorized to choose which provisions of the ACA might apply to the territories," HHS waived six major requirements – such as guaranteed issue, community rating, and essential benefit mandates – that were causing serious disruption to health insurance markets. Of course, these same requirements are causing serious disruption to health insurance markets here in the fifty states, too.

44. Failure to enforce abortion restrictions – (September 16, 2014)

A GAO report found that many exchange insurance plans don't separate charges for abortion services as required by the ACA, showing that the administration is not enforcing the law. In 2014, abortions were being financed with taxpayer funds in more than 1,000 exchange plans. (more on this in Chapter Eight)

45. Risk Corridor coverage – (September 30, 2014)

The Obama administration plans to illegally distribute risk corridor payments to insurers, despite studies by both the Congressional Research Service and the GAO saying a congressional appropriation is required before federal agencies can make the payments.

46. Transparency of coverage – (October 20, 2014)

CMS delays statutory requirements on insurance companies to disclose data on the number of people enrolled, disenrollment, number of claims denied, costs to consumers of certain services, etc.

47. Tax Penalty Pass – (February 25, 2015)

Approximately 50,000 taxpayers filed income tax returns based upon inaccurate subsidy data they received from the federal government. The administration declared that if they received too large of a subsidy, they will not have to replay the government. The ACA requires, in Section 5000A, that 'Any penalty imposed. . . shall be included with a taxpayer's return. . . '

Changes Made by Congress

These changes were made by Congress since my earlier book was written:

48. Eliminating Caps on Deductibles for Small Group Plans – (April 1, 2014)

Congress eliminated the cap on deductibles for small group plans as part of the SGR (known as the "doc fix"). This change gives small businesses the freedom to offer high deductible plans that may be paired with a Health Savings Account (HSA).

49. Making the Risk Corridor Program Budget Neutral – (December 16, 2014)

The Consolidated and Further Continuing Appropriations Act of 2015 provides that CMS may not transfer funds from other accounts to pay for the risk corridor program. Expenditures cannot exceed the funds collected in 2014, blocking CMS from making multi-year calculations.

This brings us up to date as of March, 2015. There have now been 49 changes to the law; 17 lawful changes made by Congress and two by the Supreme Court. There have been 30 *unlawful* changes made by President Obama. . . so far. (Changes chronicled by The Galen Institute)

* * *

Other Assaults on the Constitution

The litany of changes to ObamaCare is long and shameful, but this is not the only area of government that has been impacted by President Obama's assaults on the Constitution. This could be the subject of an entire book so I'll highlight only some of the most egregious examples.

NLRB Recess Appointments

The Constitution allows the President to make appointments of government officials, who would otherwise require approval by the Senate, during times when the Senate is in a period of recess.

The purpose of this authority, given by the Founding Fathers, was to allow for the appointment of those government leaders whose absence would represent a severe hardship to the operation of the government when Congress would not be in session for a long time. In those days travel was mostly by horseback and it took weeks or even months for some Senators to travel home and then return to Washington.

In modern times, however, the custom of many presidents has been to make "recess appointments" whenever the Senate *declares a recess* in order to avoid the approval process for controversial appointees. Both parties have done this in the past but until recently they respected the Senate Majority leader's right to declare when they were in recess.

However, with the growing contentiousness of Congress in recent years, the Democrats first chose a new tactic. In order to prevent President George W. Bush from making any "recess appointments" of contentious candidates, they chose to hold a series of short, minute-long pro forma sessions every three days to maintain the appearance that the Senate was still in session, not recess. President Bush respected this tactic and chose not to make any "recess appointments" during these pro forma sessions.

But President Obama chose to ignore the law and this tradition and determined on his own that the Senate was not in session. He used this excuse to appoint three very controversial candidates to the National Labor Relations Board (NLRB).

Writing in *National Review,* Josh Blackman tells us the president actually had three options when faced with the difficulty of winning approval of his nominees:

"First, he could have prevailed upon Senate Democrats to trigger the so-called nuclear option – that is, to eliminate filibustering of presidential nominations. (Two years later, Senate Majority Leader Harry Reid did just this, paving the way for confirmations with only a majority vote in the Senate.)

Second, he could have picked more palatable nominees. (A year later he did just that by withdrawing the nomination of a controversial board member and substituting an alternative whom Republicans were more willing to back.)

Third, (the option he chose) faced with a political problem that called for a political solution, the president turned to an unconstitutional shortcut: Although the Senate hadn't gone on recess – what he wanted to happen – Obama acted as if it had. During a 72 hour window between pro forma sessions on January 3 and January 6, 2012, the president deemed the Senate in recess and made three appointments to the NLRB."

Naturally, Republicans were furious and proceeded to file a lawsuit challenging the president's appointments. The issue took two years to reach the Supreme Court but when it did, *NLRB v. Noel Canning,* unanimously struck down the president's actions. All nine justices, including the two Obama appointees, specifically refuted the government's argument that gridlock in Congress justified his redefinition of the separation of powers embodied in the Constitution.

Justice Stephen Breyer, a liberal, wrote the majority opinion. He said, *"political opposition in the Senate would not qualify as an unusual circumstance"* to justify the president's making recess appointments during pro forma sessions. All nine justices concurred.

Blackman summarized the take-home message of the High Court's decision: *"The lesson from all nine justices was clear: Gridlock does not give the chief executive a license to redefine his constitutional powers."*

The government's argument, put forth by Solicitor General Donald H. Verrilli, that the president had to act because *"the NLRB was going to go dark. . . It was going to lose its quorum"* fell flat with even the liberal justices. However, it clarified Obama's rationale for all of his Executive branch over-reach. If Congress does not give him what he wants he'll find another way regardless of whether it is lawful or not.

The DREAM Act

When campaigning for the presidency, Obama promised comprehensive immigration reform if he was elected. Yet, when he had a Democratic majority in both houses of Congress in his first two years, he still failed to put forth a bill for comprehensive immigration reform.

The issue has become more contentious as his presidency has continued. The DREAM Act was proposed in Congress, which Obama endorsed, which would have provided work permits and a form of permanent residency for immigrants who were brought to the United States illegally as minors. Though the bill did gain some bipartisan support in both house of Congress, it was killed by a Republican filibuster in the Senate.

Once again, the president had several choices for his response. Blackman describes them as these:

"First - He could propose a compromise immigration policy that would receive enough support to overcome the Senate filibuster – perhaps by also strengthening border security and increasing enforcement action. But this was probably impossible.

Second - So his only practicable option was to accept a legislative defeat, which he could then use as a political issue as he campaigned against Republicans in his upcoming reelection campaign.

Third – (instead) He determined that he now had the power unilaterally to defer deportation of the immigrants in question and announced the imposition of this policy (called Deferred Action for Childhood Arrivals - DACA). Using "prosecutorial discretion," the president declared that "eligible individuals who do not present a risk to national security or public safety will be able to request temporary relief from deportation proceedings and apply for work authorization."

DACA thus accomplished the goals of the DREAM Act despite his failure to win legislative approval. This unlawful action excused over 1 million people, as a class, from the scope of Congress's naturalization powers.

President Obama responded, *"In the absence of any immigration action from Congress to fix our broken immigration system, we're improving immigration policy on our own."* In other words, if Congress won't give me what I want I'll take it on my own.

You might ask why he went to Congress for approval of the DREAM Act in the first place if he believed he had the authority to do it on his own?

Since then the issue has grown in its intensity. Republicans are now convinced that they cannot propose any acceptable immigration policy because no matter what the law will say the president will ignore those provisions of the law he disapproves. As a result House Speaker John Boehner announced in June, 2014, that the House would not bring an immigration bill to a vote this year. Gridlock would continue.

President Obama responded to this announcement with one of his own. He promptly declared he would take more unilateral actions without Congressional approval to bring about immigration reform. He said, *"I take executive action only when we have a serious problem, a serious issue, and Congress chooses to do nothing."* He would, *"fix the immigration system on my own, without Congress."*

As Justice Antonin Scalia wrote in his *NLRB v. Channing* opinion, *"gridlock is not a bug to be fixed by this Court, but a calculated feature of the constitutional framework."* In other words, if the two parties cannot agree then some sort of compromise is needed. Apparently, President Obama doesn't believe in compromise.

Religious Freedom Restrictions

We have already discussed how ObamaCare attempts to restrict our religious freedom by compelling all employers to provide health insurance that pays for contraceptives, sterilization procedures, and abortifacients. *Hobby Lobby v. Burwell* was won by the plaintiffs and secured the religious freedom of closely-held corporations and small businesses. The *non-profit* lawsuits have yet to reach the Supreme Court so that issue is still unsettled.

But the Obama administration's emphasis is clear; they believe it is more important to provide *free* contraceptives, sterilization procedures, and abortifacients than to respect the religious freedom of those Americans who object to paying for them. None of these lawsuits attempts to prevent anyone from receiving these treatments; they simply object on moral and religious grounds to being responsible for providing them.

There is another issue in this realm that speaks to the intentions of the Obama administration. That issue concerns the right of religious organizations to determine who they employ.

Hosanna-Tabor Evangelical Lutheran Church and School operates a K – 8 school founded on biblical principles. Cheryl Perich was a commissioned minister in the Church who taught fourth grade, taught religion, and led worship services. She was dismissed for insubordination and disruptive conduct and threatening to sue the Church. All of these actions are in violation of church teachings. The Church and its denomination have long taught that disputes over fitness for ministry must be resolved within the framework of the denomination.

The Becket Fund, a law firm specializing in representing Christian organizations, defended the Church when Perich brought a lawsuit. The Church argued that forcing it to retain Perich against its will, or forcing it to pay large sums of money to get rid of her would be an unconstitutional restriction on its right to choose its religious leaders.

After a victory for the church in the lower federal courts, Perich won on appeal to the Sixth Circuit Court of Appeals setting up a Supreme Court showdown. The Becket Fund web site explains the issue:

"The lower courts are unanimously agreed that ministers cannot sue their churches in disputes over qualifications, job performance, or rules for ministry – a rule known as the "ministerial exception." The federal trial court applied the ministerial exception and ruled for the Church. But the Sixth Circuit Court of Appeals held for Perich, ruling that she was just a fourth-grade teacher and not really a minister."

After appeal to the Supreme Court, the Becket Fund picks up the story:

"Perich and the Equal Employment Opportunity Commission have now escalated the dispute, arguing that there should be no ministerial exception and that any minister – even a priest, a rabbi, or a pastor of a congregation – should be able to sue the church that employs him. This would be a revolution in church-state relations."

"On January 11, 2012, the government lost 9 – 0 as the Court unanimously rejected its narrow view of religious liberty as "extreme, untenable, and remarkable." The unanimous decision adopted the Becket Fund's arguments, saying that religious groups should be free from government interference when they choose their leaders. The Court rejected the government's extremely narrow understanding of the constitutional protection for religious liberty, stating: "We cannot accept the remarkable view that the Religion Clauses have nothing to say about a religious organization's freedom to select is own ministers."

It is noteworthy that even Justice Elena Kagan, former Solicitor General and appointee by President Obama, joined in a powerful concurring opinion with Justice Antonin Scalia in rebuking the White House arguments.

It is clear from these and other cases argued before the Supreme Court that the Obama administration holds antipathy to religious freedom in this country. John Fund and Hans von Spakovsky, in a remarkable book called *Obama's Enforcer,* chronicle the abuses of the President and his Attorney General Eric Holder.

They present case after case demonstrating their pro-abortion, anti-religious ideology. They favor weakening immigration law, weakening voter-id laws, and strengthening the rights of the government over the rights of individuals. This perverse ideology is the driving force in everything the Justice Department seeks to accomplish under these two men, and they have no hesitation in trampling the Constitution to achieve their goals.

4

The Reality of Medicaid

"The evidence in the medical literature is overwhelming that Medicaid is harming most beneficiaries."
Avik Roy, Senior Fellow - The Manhattan Institute,
Forbes, 3/2/11

It is a favorite talking point of the left that the expansion of Medicaid will *"save lives."* Liberal journalist Scott Maxwell of *The Orlando Sentinel* made this exact assertion recently in a column. It's easy to see why Maxwell might believe that. Without information to verify that assumption, one would assume that giving people Medicaid insurance would improve their health and, in some cases, even save lives.

But research often refutes our sincerest assumptions. In 2008 the State of Oregon was faced with a dilemma. They wanted to expand Medicaid eligibility to more residents, but they didn't have enough money to pay for everyone. So they held a lottery for low-income, uninsured adults. This created an ideal situation for studying the impact of Medicaid in a randomized, prospective manner.

This study, known as The Oregon Health Insurance Experiment, is an ongoing study, which has already revealed significant information. Thus far, researchers have learned that having Medicaid does not improve health, at least in standard measurements of blood pressure, blood sugar, and cholesterol. Medicaid reduced observed rates of depression by 30% but increased the probability of being diagnosed with depression. Medicaid significantly increased the probability of being *diagnosed* with diabetes and the use of diabetes medication, but did not have the expected impact of *lowering* blood sugar. In other words, Medicaid had no impact on actual healthcare outcomes.

Emergency Room Usage

It has always been postulated that the uninsured are more likely to use Emergency Rooms at hospitals for their health care than the insured. By this reasoning, expansion of Medicaid would lower the use of hospital Emergency Rooms and contribute to solving this chronic problem, which poorly utilizes health care resources and increases costs. Unfortunately, the Oregon study showed the opposite. Those with newly enrolled Medicaid were *40 percent more likely* to use the Emergency Room than the uninsured. This means expanding Medicaid will actually exacerbate this problem and increase the cost of delivering health care.

A report from the Colorado Hospital Association confirms this same conclusion. In September, 2014, they reported the average number of emergency department visits to hospitals, in states that expanded Medicaid, increased 5.6% from second-quarter 2013 to second-quarter 2014. This change was greater than expected from the variation over the last two years, resulting in the highest number of average visits over that time. In comparison, hospitals in non-expansion states reported only a 1.8% increase in emergency department visits in the same period.

John R. Graham, writing for *The National Center for Policy Analysis,* notes this shows Medicaid expansion increased E R visits three times as much compared to states without Medicaid expansion. While this report may be welcomed by hospitals looking for more government revenue to compensate for non-paying customers, it bodes poorly for those with Medicaid.

Why do Medicaid patients use the emergency room more? John C. Goodman, founder of *The National Center for Policy Analysis*, explains this in his book, *Priceless.* Goodman says having Medicaid may actually be worse than having no insurance at all. That's because most doctors do not accept Medicaid patients and the ones who do often ration their appointments making waiting times very long. Medicaid patients respond by going to the Emergency Room where they are sure to be seen the same day.

The uninsured actually have greater *access* to health care. They can see practically any physician any time by negotiating a discounted cash rate that will still pay the doctor more than Medicaid. The result is less need to use Emergency Rooms for primary care. Medicaid patients are barred by law from paying doctors more than Medicaid allows.

Most people assume that you have to have health care insurance to get good health care. But this assumption has been disproven by multiple studies. A RAND Corporation study found virtually no difference in the quality of care received by the insured and the uninsured among people *who seek care*. In a thorough study of the impact of health insurance, former Clinton adviser Richard Kronick found that insurance had virtually no effect on mortality. The uninsured *who seek care* can usually find quality care.

There are more perverse outcomes from having Medicaid. Avik Roy, health care blogger for *Forbes* magazine, has reported the following studies:

- A University of Virginia study found that individuals enrolled in Medicaid are almost twice as likely to die after surgery as privately insured patients, and about one-eighth more likely to die *than the uninsured!*
- A study published in the *Journal of the National Cancer Institute* found that Florida Medicaid patients were 6 percent more likely to be diagnosed with prostate cancer at less treatable, later stages than the uninsured. Medicaid enrollees were nearly one-third more likely to be diagnosed with late-stage breast cancer and 81 percent more likely to be diagnosed with melanoma at a late stage than the uninsured.

- A study in the journal *Cancer* found that the mortality rate for Medicaid patients undergoing surgery for colon cancer was more than three times as high as for the privately insured and more than one-fourth higher than for the uninsured
- A study in the *Journal of Vascular Surgery* found that Medicaid patients treated for vascular problems, including plaque in their carotid arteries and femoral arteries, fared worse than did the uninsured.

These are not the only studies Roy has found that lead him to conclude that Medicaid patients do no better, and sometimes worse, than the uninsured.

It seems that many in the Medicaid eligible population have figured this out. A report in *The New England Journal of Medicine* by Sommers and Epstein states that there are over nine million Americans eligible for Medicaid who are currently *not enrolled.* They could have Medicaid at any time just by signing up but for various reasons they have failed to do so. Undoubtedly, some of the reasons include the inconveniences of enrollment, the long waiting times on telephones or in government offices. But some have already concluded, rightly, they may be better off without insurance at all.

The University of Virginia Study

Skeptics on the left have challenged the conclusions of Roy, especially concerning the University of Virginia (UVa) Study. So let's take a moment to look deeper at the conclusions of the authors of the study themselves.

First of all, this was a landmark study. The research team of doctors at UVa looked at surgical operations from 2003 to 2007, a five-year analysis. The study included 893,658 major surgical procedures. This represents an enormous number of patients and surgical procedures. The patients were stratified by primary payer status, on three outcomes endpoints: in-hospital mortality, length of stay, and total costs incurred. The authors state this study, "*represents the largest and most comprehensive analysis of surgical outcomes by insurance status ever conducted."*

Second, the authors normalized the results for age, gender, income, geographic region, operation, and 30 background diseases. These adjustments are made to eliminate bias in the study's conclusions. The authors summarize their findings:

"Our results indicate that Medicaid and Uninsured payer status confers worse unadjusted and adjusted outcomes compared with that of Private Insurance. We have shown that Medicaid and Uninsured status also independently increase the risk of adjusted in-hospital mortality, and that complications compared with those with Private Insurance.

Moreover, our results demonstrate significant differences in resource utilization among payer groups as Medicaid patients accrued the longest adjusted hospital length of stay and highest adjusted total costs. These findings bolster those of other smaller series that have been performed in select surgical populations, and it extends the examination of payer status to include a large, nationwide, diverse surgical population."

To the argument that this represents only one study, the authors also note similar findings in studies by Giacovelli et al (2008) and Kelz et al (2004).

In reviewing the landmark work of these authors, Roy draws the following conclusions:

*"Patients on Medicare were 45% more likely to die than those with private insurance; the uninsured were 74% more likely; and Medicaid patients 93% more likely. That is to say, despite the fact that we will soon spend more than $500 Billion a year on Medicaid, Medicaid beneficiaries, on average, **fared worse than those with no insurance at all."***

Roy calls this, *"the greatest scandal in America. Bigger than Madoff, bigger than the Wall Street bailout, bigger even than the plight of the uninsured."*

Medicaid Expansion

Despite these ominous conclusions about Medicaid, ObamaCare actually seeks to expand Medicaid. In fact, the original goal was to increase Medicaid enrollment by about 15 million Americans. The Obama administration will never achieve this goal, however, because they lost their bid in the Supreme Court to compel the states to accept Medicaid expansion or lose all Medicaid federal funding (Chapter Two). The result is only half the states have accepted the expansion of Medicaid.

The Obama administration never expected this outcome. The law was written with strong incentives for states to comply with expansion. It calls for 100% federal support of the increased cost of Medicaid expansion for the first three years, declining to 90% thereafter. But just to be sure the states complied, they provided in the statute for denial of all federal funding of Medicaid if states objected to expansion. The Supreme Court held this portion of the law unconstitutional.

Despite the incentives, many governors are more concerned about the future cost of Medicaid expansion and prudently declined this federal offer. They already will have to bear the burden of increasing Medicaid enrollment of those un-enrolled by the old eligibility standards. The states will have to pay for these new enrollees by the current federal subsidies, which average only 57 percent of the costs. These costs could be substantial in some states like Florida and Texas where current enrollment is less than 50 percent of those eligible.

New Democratic Virginia Governor Terry McAuliffe recently tried to force Medicaid expansion down the throats of his Republican majority House of Representatives. He insisted the expansion would create 30,000 jobs and save the state over $1 billion over eight years. But there is no evidence to prove these claims. In fact, expansion is more likely to cost the state billions.

Fred Barnes, writing in *The Wall Street Journal,* tells the reasons for the opposition of the Republican Speaker of the House, William Howell:

"Under ObamaCare, the federal government would pay 100% of the Medicaid expansion for three years, then 90% until 2022. Mr. Howell estimates the expansion will cost Virginia $40 million to $50 million in administrative expenses even when Washington supposedly is paying 100%. When that dips to 90%, another $200 million to $250 million will be added to the state's annual tab."

Governor McAuliffe has threatened to take unilateral action without the legislature's approval (much like his close ally, President Obama). However, Mr. Howell countered by hiring prominent constitutional lawyer Paul Clement to assess the legality of such a move. Clement's response was blunt: *"No funds may be expended to finance any attempt by the Governor to expand Medicaid unilaterally."*

This clearly illustrates the financial barriers to expansion of Medicaid by the states. The cost of Medicaid currently averages 25% or more of most state budgets, exceeded only by education. Any state legislature exercising fiscal discipline should be wary of Medicaid expansion under the terms of ObamaCare.

Medicaid for Children

To be fair, there is some evidence to suggest that children may still benefit from Medicaid over being uninsured. Studies show the pediatric population is different from the adult population. Due to the fragility of infants and children, especially if they are lacking a parent, any care, no matter how bad, is probably still better than none at all. Children must receive antibiotics and vaccinations to avoid the numerous diseases that plague childhood. These are relatively cheap and easy to provide and can make a substantial difference.

The benefits of Medicaid decline with increasing income and age. Based on data that is between 20 and 30 years old, Medicaid may benefit the very poorest children as well as their mothers during pregnancy. It is unclear if this data will hold up with a more recent study.

ObamaCare seeks to expand Medicaid coverage of the uninsured but doesn't provide the means to increase *access* to health care.

Without *access* to health care, any insurance is just a piece of paper; as useless as a discount coupon for bottled water to a man wandering in the desert. Unless you can *access* the health care you need you will be no better off than you were before.

A recent study published in the Orthopedic literature illustrates the problem. Researchers at The University of North Carolina devised fictional patients with orthopedic problems and described scenarios that implied the need for urgent surgery within two weeks. Then they surveyed 203 orthopedic practices in the state of North Carolina requesting an appointment within two weeks for these fictional patients.

The survey was taken in two parts. The first part described the patient as having Medicaid insurance. The second part, taken three weeks later, described the same patient scenario but with private health insurance. The only variable in the two fictional patients was their type of insurance.

In the first part, patients with Medicaid insurance were offered an appointment within two weeks 59 percent of the calls. In the second part, patients with private insurance were offered an appointment within two weeks 79 percent of the calls. Clearly, patients with Medicaid face a greater barrier to access of medical care when compared to those patients with private health insurance.

The study showed this barrier to access of healthcare gets worse in more populous areas and in areas closer to academic medical centers. It gets better in less populous areas and in areas more distant from academic medical centers. Practices more than 60 miles from academic hospitals were more likely to accept patients with Medicaid than practices closer to academic hospitals.

So *access* to specialty care gets worse when there is an abundance of such care in the community.

In fact, ObamaCare will probably *decrease access* since an increased volume of patients will not be accompanied by an increased source of providers. There are no provisions in the law to increase the training of doctors or other health care providers.

Goodman explains how ObamaCare will actually *decrease access* to health- care in three ways:

- The major barrier to care for low-income families is the same in the United States as it is throughout the developed world: *the time price of care* and other non-price rationing mechanisms are far more important than the money price of care.
- The burdens of non-price rationing rise as income falls, with the lowest-income families facing the longest waiting times and the largest bureaucratic obstacles to care.
- ObamaCare, by lowering the out-of-pocket money price of care for almost everybody while doing nothing to change supply, will intensify non-price rationing and may actually make access to care more difficult for those with the least financial resources.

In other words, price is not the most important barrier to healthcare; long waiting times to see a doctor are. This "non-price rationing", in the words of an economist, gets worse for those with the least financial resources. *This means ObamaCare will actually make getting health care more difficult for those the law was most intended to help.*

Medicaid Reform

Therefore, the obvious question is, "How can we improve Medicaid? There are many ideas that have been put forth already. Before we discuss some of them, however, we need to understand what's right and wrong with Medicaid.

If an insurance company came out with a new product that promised to provide health care with no deductibles, no co-payments, no primary care approvals, no limits on coverage, *and no premiums to pay,* you would probably say, "It's too good to be true." Yet that's exactly what Medicaid looks like – on paper. It is free to those who qualify, does not require deductibles or co-pays, has no ceilings, and doesn't require approvals. But nobody wants it.

The reason is simple. The fees paid to doctors are so low that few doctors will accept this insurance. How low are they? Medicaid pays hospitals and doctors less than 60 percent of what private insurers pay.

In fact, studies now show that Medicaid pays only 70% of the *overhead costs* of providing doctors' services - Medicare is only slightly better at 78%. *That means doctors lose money every time they treat a Medicaid or Medicare patient.* No wonder few doctors accept Medicaid and only slightly more accept Medicare.

Those doctors that do accept Medicaid usually practice a routine of restricting the number of Medicaid appointments so that better-paying patients are seen first. The result is long waits for an appointment even from those who will accept Medicaid. Medicaid patients figure this out quickly and respond by using hospital emergency rooms for their primary care needs even though the waiting times there can be several hours. At least they know they'll be seen sometime the same day.

The solution to this problem seems obvious. Pay the doctors more – at least enough to cover their overhead! There is no question this would help solve the problem, but the political challenge of finding the funds to pay for this is a more daunting task. So let's talk about other solutions.

Suggested Solutions

My suggestion is to let the patients pay more. This may seem obvious, but it is really more complicated.

First, you must change the laws governing Medicaid (and Medicare) that prohibit the doctors from accepting higher payment from the patients than these programs pay. Today an uninsured patient can go into nearly any doctor's office and negotiate a discounted fee-for-service rate to see the doctor. Discounts may be as much as 50% off for cash patients. But Medicaid (and Medicare) patients are prohibited by law from making any similar arrangements with their doctors.

If the laws are changed, I suggest letting patients negotiate with their doctors to pay slightly more than Medicaid pays. Some doctors would agree to accept a10% co-pay above what Medicaid pays; others would accept 20% or more. Doctors could even advertise their rates to attract more Medicaid patients – which they would do if the fees were higher.

Many Medicaid patients would gladly pay 10 or 20% more to avoid the long waiting times at hospital emergency rooms. The beauty of this solution is there would be no increase in the cost to the taxpayers. This should gain bipartisan support in Congress.

Florida

There are other solutions to Medicaid. Former Florida Governor Jeb Bush initiated a pilot program in 2006 in five counties with a population of nearly three million people and a Medicaid population of 290,000. These Medicaid enrollees were allowed to choose among competing, private managed-care plans, with varying provider networks and benefit packages as long as they cover mandatory benefits. Also, enrollees were given incentives to manage their own health and to encourage healthy behavior.

Five years later the results of this study showed higher patient satisfaction at a lower cost than traditional Medicaid. These programs offer better care and *access* to specialists has improved. One estimate is that this pilot program is saving $161 million per year for the state of Florida. Imagine if this were multiplied by the remaining counties in Florida and the other 49 states! One estimate is that the program would save $91 billion annually while improving health outcomes and achieving enrollee satisfaction scores of 83 to 100 percent.

Indiana

The State of Indiana has also tried new innovations in Medicaid. In 2007, Indiana Governor Mitch Daniels established The Healthy Indiana Plan to provide low-income families with consumer-driven health plans, coupled with personal health accounts called a Power Account. The purpose was not only to boost health coverage but also to encourage enrollees to take a more active role in their health care decisions.

Those low-income families uninsured for six months or longer were enrolled in the program but asked to make monthly contributions of 2 to 5 percent of their income (up to $92). The state contributed $1100 to the account, which covers nearly three-quarters of the deductible. Preventive care is covered by the plan on a first-dollar basis (no cost to patient). Once the $1500 deductible is met there are no other costs to the patients.

About 45,000 Indianans participated in the program and 90 percent made their contributions. Satisfaction was measured at 98 percent. However, the Obama administration decided not to renew the federal waiver required to continue the program.

National Center for Policy Analysis

John C. Goodman of the National Center for Policy Analysis has other ideas. One would be to abolish Medicaid entirely and use the money instead to subsidize the integration of poor patients into the same healthcare system everyone else uses. He proposes refundable health insurance tax credits of $2000/person and $8000/family of four. These would not be cash payments but rather a voucher for purchasing health insurance. With these vouchers, low-income families could purchase health insurance from traditional private insurers. Just in case you're worried that wouldn't be enough, he suggests keeping traditional Medicaid available until the private market proves they can do better. He thinks most people would choose the private alternative.

Goodman has other ideas. He proposes a "Health Stamp" program patterned after the food stamp (SNAP) program currently in use for purchasing food for low-income families. This would empower these families to purchase their health care on a level playing field with other patients. Just as those who purchase their food with food stamps do so in the same grocery stores as other consumers, these families would purchase their health care from the same doctors and hospitals that accept traditional insurance.

There are over 60 million Americans currently purchasing their food with food stamps. They are welcome in every grocery store because their stamps are as good as cash. They make their purchases based on the limits of their resources but the prices are transparent and therefore they can make informed decisions. They can spend more of their own money if they can afford it. The same would be true of health stamps. This would insure that the poor could compete for health care resources with all other buyers of care.

All of these proposals would improve *access* to health care for low-income families. They all level the playing field for the poor by reducing or eliminating the disparity in physician payments between Medicaid patients and other patients. Doctors don't discriminate against Medicaid patients because they don't like them; they discriminate because their time is unequally compensated in our traditional Medicaid system. Doctors, like all business owners, must make sure they can pay their bills if they are to continue providing health care for anyone. A level playing field for the poor would insure that Medicaid patients would be just as welcome in doctor's offices as all other patients.

The Apothecary

Avik Roy, healthcare blogger for *The Apothecary,* suggests another approach. He believes we should approach the problem much as Switzerland does. They allow the poor to obtain private insurance and control their own healthcare spending. This would be possible through tax credits, established by means-testing, which would give the poor subsidies to purchase health insurance in the private insurance market.

In this respect, it would mimic ObamaCare. However, he would do away with the Individual and Employer Mandates and the "community rating" that makes ObamaCare so expensive. Community rating drives the cost of health insurance up for everyone and forces the poor to purchase low quality insurance policies on the exchanges.

Roy's solution would eliminate Medicaid as we know it (and maybe Medicare, too) and put everyone in a private insurance policy.

This would level the playing field so that low-income Americans would not feel they are being treated differently and would go a long way toward improving access to healthcare.

Improved *access* to care would then achieve improved health care outcomes. That should be our real goal in reforming health care; not just expanding the number of people with health insurance.

Roy further suggests that if you do not eliminate Medicaid then it should be converted to a system of block grants to the states. That way the federal government would give the states free rein to compare market-oriented and socialized approaches to Medicaid; and see which ones work best.

The Hill

There are others who agree. Antos, Capretta, Doar, and Pauly, writing for *The Hill,* make similar recommendations. First, they call for a universal tax credit for any household without access to employer-financed insurance, including Medicaid participants. They believe this subsidy should be sufficient to ensure that all Americans can purchase private insurance protection against large medical expenses.

Second, they believe states must have the flexibility to use Medicaid's resources more effectively. Medicaid should be converted into premium support for insurance, and participants should be able to select their own insurance plan – including an employer plan, if one is available.

Third, they call for investments in better health clinics to catch those who fall between the cracks. They want a new approach to rely on competitive bidding to select the most cost-effective approaches for improving the health status of poor households. They conclude:

"Providing a secure and accessible health system for the poor will not occur without some public expense, and will require additional discipline elsewhere in the budget. But that should not be an excuse for failing to reform a dysfunctional system."

ObamaCare's Impact on Medicaid

As we have discussed earlier, ObamaCare hoped to expand Medicaid by about 15 million newly enrolled Americans. The Supreme Court struck down the involuntary expansion of Medicaid by the states and made it voluntary. Therefore, Medicaid has not expanded as much as the Obama administration desired.

Nevertheless, Medicaid enrollment has substantially increased. In fact, a new report by the Urban Institute states the increased coverage of the uninsured by ObamaCare is largely an expansion of Medicaid (70%). This has broad implications for the future of healthcare reform.

More people will have Medicaid insurance, but with less access to health care, at an increasing cost to the federal and state governments, with no real measurable improvement in their physical health. This is a formula for medical and fiscal disaster, not a solution to the problems of our health care system and our financial future. We must find solutions that better address the need for *access* to health care in ways that will not bankrupt the nation or the states.

5

The Insurance Bailout Has Begun

"The non-surprise revealed here is that ObamaCare turns out to be just another subsidy program, throwing money at health care."
Holman W. Jenkins, Jr.
The Wall Street Journal, 9/16/14

Insurance companies are rarely the objects of sympathy. Most people, especially doctors like me, spend much too much time and money battling with insurance companies to get paid what they owe us. We all know the basic insurance business model is taking our money and then holding onto it as long as possible, even when they are responsible to pay for covered expenses.

Yet some have actually suggested they are losers in the new health care law, ObamaCare, because they must provide expensive benefits and accept patients without actuarial risk adjustment. Some even suggest they may be out of business soon.

It is true that insurance companies have been forced to change their usual way of doing business in ways that force them to accept higher risks for patients with pre-existing diseases. ObamaCare forces them to use "community rating" to determine their premium prices rather than sound actuarial analysis of risk. Rather than calculate the true cost of covering these individuals, insurance companies can only vary the cost by age, tobacco usage, and geographical location of residence. They are not allowed to deny coverage to anyone because of pre-existing medical conditions.

Also, the usual six levels of insurance premium prices, based on risk factors, have been reduced to three. The result is high-risk patients pay less than usual while low-risk patients, especially the young, pay much more.

For these reasons there has been greater attention paid to the number of new enrollees in ObamaCare and a greater scrutiny of the age and pre-existing medical conditions of the enrollees. The concern is an insufficient number of new enrollees, especially in the young and healthy demographic of 18 – 34 year-olds, will leave the insurance companies with higher costs and less revenue. This may lead to a so-called "death spiral" for insurance companies that forces them to raise prices to compensate for losses – which will further decrease the number of new enrollees.

But, have no fear. You, the taxpayers, are near.

The "Three Rs"

ObamaCare has provisions in the law to protect the insurance companies – not the taxpayers. In order to ensure the cooperation of the insurance companies, the authors of this law (not Congress – they never read it) inserted three methods of bailing out the insurance companies.

Jay Cost and Jeffrey H. Anderson, writing in *The Weekly Standard*, call these the "Three Rs" – *risk adjustment, reinsurance,* and *risk corridors*. These three provisions in the law were sufficient enticements to guarantee the compliance of the insurance industry in this makeover of our healthcare delivery system.

Risk adjustment spreads the wealth around from those insurance companies with relatively healthy enrollees to those with sicker enrollees who cost more to insure. This compensates for the loss of the right to refuse those with pre-existing expensive medical conditions and the unsound actuarial pricing ObamaCare requires. If your company happens to get stuck with too many sick patients and not enough healthy ones, the risk adjustment provisions in the law will compensate for your losses.

Reinsurance is actually a tax added to the price of every health insurance policy of $63/person for the next three years. Most Americans will pay this tax except certain unions that have received exemptions from the Obama administration as a political payback for their election support. That's one of many changes to the law that President Obama made without Congressional approval.

This provision, described in Section 1341 of the Affordable Care Act, is expected to raise about $25 Billion by the year 2016. This money will flow to the insurance companies to allow them to hold down future premium prices that would otherwise skyrocket under ObamaCare. In reality, what these funds do is subsidize the premiums paid on the ObamaCare exchanges out of higher premium policies paid by those receiving their insurance through employers.

Risk corridors, described in Section 1342 of the ACA, are also designed to prop up the insurance companies in case their expenses exceed their revenues. Insurance industry consultant Robert Laszewski explains that if an insurance company expects its costs in a given year to be X, and those costs end up being more than X plus 2 percent, taxpayers will come to that insurance company's rescue. Once an insurance company covers that initial 2 percent cost overage, taxpayers will cover at least 80 percent of any additional costs the insurer accrues.

The Three Rs were intended to stabilize the insurance market until there were enough enrollees to guarantee the financial stability of the insurers. This was all predicated on the expectation that people would like ObamaCare and would sign up for it in record numbers; or at least they would enroll because of the tax called The Individual Mandate, which assesses a tax upon any individual who does not have health insurance by 2014.

However, the botched rollout of the government web site Healthcare.gov, and the increasing public awareness of the problems with ObamaCare, have contributed to lower than expected enrollment. Furthermore, once again President Obama has delayed the impact of the Individual Mandate, without Congressional approval, and thereby threatened the financial stability of the insurance industry. This will contribute to the need for earlier bailout of the insurance companies than expected.

Also influential are the numerous delays to the ACA unilaterally determined by the White House in response to the rising tide of criticism of the law. They recognized the growing reality that the law was a political albatross for those Democrats seeking re-election to Congress in November 2014. Obama has grandfathered existing health plans in some cases, delayed the Employer Mandate, and even watered down the requirements for compliance with the Individual Mandate to the point where it is functionally irrelevant. All of these decisions have been made to protect vulnerable Congressional Democrats, but all have contributed to the increased necessity of a taxpayer bailout of the insurance industry.

Another ObamaCare Change

Cost and Anderson write that May 16, 2014, the administration finalized adjustments to two of the programs – *reinsurance* and *risk corridors* – to funnel more money to insurers. They lowered the threshold at which insurers become eligible for reinsurance money, and made more generous the formula by which insurers get paid under the risk corridors. This represented the 42nd change to ObamaCare since the law was passed in 2010 and the 25th unlawful change made unilaterally by President Obama (see Chapter Three).

Seth Chandler, a University of Houston law professor with a background in insurance law, writes, *"It's an extremely sneaky way of sending money to the insurance industry, resting, as it does, on arcane manipulations of mathematical formulae. And I have serious doubts that the changes are authorized by Congress."*

According to the non-partisan Congressional Budget Office (CBO) these changes are estimated to cost taxpayers an additional $8 Billion. The original expectation of the risk corridors was projected to *generate $8 Billion in revenue* for the government to fund the program. Now they are projected to be budget-neutral. Effectively, this means the insurance industry has just received an $8 Billion tax break – funded by the taxpayers. To put this in perspective, the Fortune 500 showed, in the year before Obama was elected, the nations' 10 largest health insurers made $8 Billion in *combined* profits.

The bad news is things could get worse. If enrollment in the ObamaCare exchanges declines as insurance premiums increase, the bailout of the insurance industry will grow. There is nothing in the ACA to require the risk corridors to be budget-neutral. The CBO has specifically addressed this concern with the following statement:

"In contrast to the risk adjustment and reinsurance programs, payments and collections under the risk corridor program will not necessarily equal one another: If insurers' costs exceed their expectations, on average, the risk corridor program will impose costs on the federal budget; if, however, insurers' costs fall below their expectations, on average, the risk corridor program will generate savings for the federal budget."

While there is little disagreement that the risk corridor program does not have to be budget-neutral, there is certainly disagreement about whether the administration has the legal authority to pay extra money to insurers (or even to pay insurers at all under the program) in the absence of a congressional appropriation. The non-partisan Congressional Research Service (CRS), in a memo dated 1/23/14, wrote, *"federal agencies are prohibited from making payments in the absence of a valid appropriation."* They opined the risk corridor language in ObamaCare *"would not appear to constitute an appropriation."*

But HHS disagrees. They assert, *"Regardless of the balance of payments and receipts, HHS will remit payments as required under . . . the Affordable Care Act."* In other words, with or without Congress.

A Slush Fund

It may be reasonably argued that the Three Rs were necessary to ensure the cooperation of the insurance industry in order to provide health insurance under ObamaCare. Notwithstanding other alternatives that are better, this argument may be valid. But what is disturbing is the use of the Three Rs to back up the lawlessness of the Obama administration changes to the ACA – which have clearly been politically motivated.

As Cost and Anderson conclude in their article, the Three Rs have effectively become a *slush fund* for the president – one that enables him to make changes to the law that suit his political agenda without destroying the insurance industry and losing their support. The only ones adversely affected are the taxpayers.

There are solutions to this problem. Charles Krauthammer, highly respected syndicated columnist of *The Washington Post,* suggested one in January. He proposed The No Bailout for Insurance Companies Act of 2014. He said it could be a one-line bill. *"Sections 1341 and 1342 of The Affordable Care Act are hereby repealed."* He succinctly put it this way, *"End of bill. End of bailout. End of story."*

Senator Marco Rubio (R – FL) has put forth a more recent solution. He has introduced in the Senate, and Rep. Leonard Lance (R – N.J.) has introduced in the House, short, simple bills requiring ObamaCare's risk corridor program to be budget-neutral. This would effectively dry up Obama's slush fund.

Only if the president intends to continue his unilateral changes in the law to suit his political agenda will he insist upon keeping the risk corridor program flexible enough to bail out the insurance industry whenever he chooses. The American taxpayer deserves better.

The Public Response

Sadly, most Americans are not paying attention to crucial issues like these. But when they are informed, the reactions are predictable.

McLaughlin and Associates, in a poll commissioned by The 2017 Project, asked likely voters, *"If private insurance companies lose money selling health insurance under ObamaCare, should taxpayers help cover their losses?* The response was overwhelming – 81% said no and only 10% said yes.

Unfortunately, at this writing, the House has not taken a vote on this issue. Clearly it would be popular with the American people. It would also establish the connection between the White House and the insurance industry. Any attempt by the White House to defeat the bill would highlight their allegiance to the insurance companies at the expense of the taxpayers.

Jeffrey H. Anderson discovered this allegiance was made clear by some recent e-mails found by the House Oversight Committee. They discovered the cozy alliance between the Obama White House and insurance companies. He writes: *"Chris Jennings, Obama's deputy assistant for health policy, coached Florida Blue Cross and Blue Shield CEO Patrick Geraghty in advance of his appearances on the CBS Evening News and Meet the Press last fall, and then emailed Geraghty afterward to exclaim, "Pat: You were extraordinary. . . We were all impressed. Thank you so much! Would like to talk soon."*

He also found the main lobbying group for the insurance companies, America's Health Insurance Plans, wrote to the administration, *"Risk corridors should be operated without the constraint of budget neutrality."* Operating them *"without the constraint of budget neutrality"* means using them to funnel taxpayer money to insurers.

Anderson says fighting the bailout – whether by repealing the risk corridors or requiring them to be budget-neutral – would help rebut one of the few remaining weapons in the Democrats' arsenal as they try to defend ObamaCare. It seems that Democrats argue Republicans are in favor of putting the insurance companies back in charge of our healthcare. They say Republicans favor big business, the insurance companies, over the people.

By bringing this issue to a vote the Republicans would expose the Democratic alliance with the insurance companies. A vote against such a bill to correct this problem would make it obvious to the people that Democrats really favor the Big Insurance lobby over the American taxpayer.

It would also be one more way to strike back at the president's lawlessness in changing ObamaCare without Congressional approval. He has made it clear from the beginning that he believes he can change the law whenever it suits his political agenda. A vote to restore the integrity of the law would strengthen Congress's powers as outlined in the Constitution.

There is more evidence of malfeasance by the White House. Holman W. Jenkins, Jr., writing in *The Wall Street Journal,* says emails last April confirm that Chet Burrell, head of Maryland insurer CareFirst, wrote to Valerie Jarrett, Obama consigliore. He complained after the administration publicly stated its "risk corridor" plan would be revenue neutral – i.e., no extra taxpayer dollars would be available to cover insurer losses. He warned her that sticking with this plan would mean politically "an unwelcome surprise," namely premium hikes of 20% or more later this year as ObamaCare policies come up for renewal.

Jarrett responded with assurances that insurers would get 80% of what they sought. Then later, the figure was tweaked in May to be closer to 100%. Without Congressional approval, any increased payments would be unlawful and increase the burden for taxpayers. But that is exactly what happened. The impact is predictable, despite Jarrett's attempts to delay the inevitable.

Jenkins says this reveals what comes as no surprise to anyone – ObamaCare turns out to be just another subsidy program, throwing money at health care. He sums up the situation thus:

"In economics, you can't subsidize everybody but we're trying: 50 million Americans get help from Medicare, 65 million from Medicaid, nine million from the Department of Veterans affairs, seven million (and counting) from ObamaCare, and a whopping 149 million from the giant tax handout for employer-provided health insurance.

Much of this money (which will total about $1.3 Trillion in 2014) is shoveled out regardless of need, driving up prices and spurring production of services of dubious value. The spending is less effective at improving the nation's health. An "Affordable Care Act" worth its title would have gotten us off this kamikaze mission. It didn't."

The Coming Train Wreck

The ObamaCare train wreck is still coming. Don't take my word for it! Even though my last book, *The ObamaCare Train Wreck,* uses this same metaphor, I can't take credit for the idea.

Credit for the original idea goes to Senator Max Baucus, Chairman of the Senate Finance Committee, in a hearing on 4/17/13 when he responded to HHS Secretary Kathleen Sebelius by saying, *"I just see a huge train wreck coming."* Sebelius was describing her preparations for the coming implementation of the Affordable Care Act on October 1, 2013. Even though he was one of the principle architects of ObamaCare and largely responsible for guiding it through Senate confirmation, he could clearly anticipate problems. Senator Baucus probably had no idea just how prescient his words would be.

As I said in Chapter One, the White House prematurely celebrated the announcement of 7.1 million Americans "signed-up" for ObamaCare. But as I have discussed in that chapter, that number is greatly inflated.

There was optimism then, and there remains optimism now among supporters of the law, that the train wreck Senator Baucus predicted will never happen. It could be argued it already happened in the failed rollout of the law when Healthcare.gov was crashing almost daily. But since the end of the open enrollment period on March 31, 2014, there has been less news about ObamaCare thereby giving the false impression that the train wreck has been averted.

But now comes an assessment of the situation nearly 17 months later by insurance expert Robert Laszewski that sounds much like that of Senator Baucus. Laszewski is a highly respected consultant to the health insurance industry who writes a popular healthcare blog. After a quiet summer with little news on ObamaCare, he predicted a different autumn with the second open enrollment period.

False Hope

Supporters of ObamaCare trumpeted the modest insurance rate increases leaked to the public in advance of the November open enrollment. They believed these are evidence that ObamaCare is working. But Laszewski explains this was predictable – and no reason for optimism.

"The 2015 rate increases have been largely modest. Does that prove ObamaCare is sustainable? No. You might recall that on this blog months ago my 2015 rate increase prediction was for increases of 9.9%.

You might also recall my reason for predicting such a modest increase. With almost no valid claims data yet and the "3Rs" ObamaCare reinsurance program, insurers have little if any useful information yet on which to base 2015 rates and the reinsurance program virtually protects the carrier from losing any money through 2016. I've actually had reports of actuarial consultants going around to the plans that failed to gain substantial market share suggesting they lower their rates in order to grab market share because they have nothing to lose with the now unlimited (the administration took the lid on payments off this summer) ObamaCare reinsurance program covering their losses."

Nevertheless, the Kaiser Family Foundation reported that average premiums will decline slightly for the Silver baseline plans in 16 markets. Rather than evidence that ObamaCare is bringing down rates, Laszewski says this merely reflects a perverse market where losing money to gain market share is good business.

"The new 2015 Silver baseline plan may have a lower premium than the 2014 Silver baseline plan. But that is almost always because the insurance company that held that slot in 2014, and almost always got the largest share of business, significantly increased their rates for 2015. Then another insurance company, who didn't write much business and likely now eager to increase market share, decreased their rates and has become the 2015 baseline plan. The second company was able to decrease their rates without much fear because the ObamaCare "3Rs" reinsurance scheme virtually protects them from any material losses.

*So, this headline about the baseline plans decreasing their rates in so many markets is more about the carriers who sold the most in the first year increasing their rates while the plans that sold very little business, and able to fall back on the ObamaCare reinsurance scheme, **cut their rates in a no-lose attempt to gain business**."*

He says the real ObamaCare insurance rates won't be known until we see the 2017 rates – when there will be adequate claims data to do accurate actuarial analysis – *and when the reinsurance program will have ended.* Until then the premium rates will be artificially supported by the Obama administration – which means the taxpayers.

Unfortunately, there is no guarantee the "3Rs" will actually end in 2016 as the law directs. Given the inclination of President Obama to change the law as it suits his political agenda, there is at least an even chance he will change the law again before that time to benefit Democrats in the 2016 elections. That would mean more artificial support of insurance rates beyond the end of his term of office – again at the expense of the American taxpayers.

More Bad News

The news gets worse. Laszewski says the government web site is still not working as needed. The HealthCare.gov backroom is not built yet – a year and counting after it should have been. This means there is still not a government-to-insurance company accounting system built so accurate numbers of enrollments are still not available. It also means that government verification of eligibility for subsidies is still not possible, either.

The HHS plan is for those currently enrolled to auto-renew their existing ObamaCare policies. They are telling people their policies will automatically renew, without the need to go to the web site to re-enroll. But Laszewski warns this could be disastrous for individuals. Once again he explains:

"The biggest reason is that in most cases the baseline second lowest cost Silver plan, upon which their personal subsidy is based,

has changed and with it the subsidy they are eligible for. The only way a participant will know the impact of price changes in their community's baseline plan on their own net of subsidy premium is to re-enroll. If they do not, they could be surprised by a big jump in their 2015 out-of-pocket premium come January, or a big tax bill a year later. And, if their income data is not up-to-date, they could be getting a much smaller or bigger subsidy than they are entitled to."

As Laszewski predicted, more confusion occurred after the November open enrollment period when people received renewal notices and cancellation letters in October for pre-ObamaCare policies no longer available. Furthermore, accurate enrollment numbers are impossible since many people will be counted by both their old insurance policy and their new one – until they fail to make the premium payments on the old policy for 90 days. Add to that the fragility of the HealthCare.gov web site, the lack of adequate security measures, as well as rising deductibles for 2015 (those go up with cost trend as well as the rates), and you have the conditions once again for a train wreck.

Socialized Medicine

"Socialized medicine is snake oil."
Charlie Reese
Orlando Sentinel columnist, 1978

It is well known that leading Democrats favor the socialized models of health care. No less than President Obama, Senate Minority Leader Harry Reid, and House Minority Leader Nancy Pelosi, are all on record as favoring single-payer or socialized medicine systems. They have admitted they would have pushed such a program for the United States if it were politically feasible when reforming our health care system during the debate in Congress in 2009 and 2010.

Evidence of their proclivity for socialized medicine is the Obama nomination of Tom Daschle, an outspoken advocate of Britain's socialized National Health Service (NHS), for the position of Health and Human Services Secretary in 2009. Daschle, the former Senate Majority Leader, failed the nomination process when he was criticized for non-payment of taxes. Instead, Kathleen Sebelius was nominated, another proponent of socialized medicine. Another advocate of the Britain NHS, Donald Berwick, was appointed interim director of the Centers for Medicare and Medicaid Services.

If you looked only at the report of the Commonwealth Fund, a private foundation focused on health care, you might think they were on the right track. Commonwealth issued a report this summer ranking the NHS as the best medical system among those in eleven of the world's most advanced nations, including Canada, France, Germany, Switzerland and Sweden. They ranked the United States last of the eleven.

But statistics can be misleading, as Dr. Scott W. Atlas of the Hoover Institution points out in a *Wall Street Journal* article. He says the Commonwealth rankings are contradicted by objective data about access and medical-care quality in peer-reviewed academic journals.

For instance, Americans diagnosed with heart disease receive treatment with medications significantly more frequently than patients in Western Europe, according to Kenneth Thorpe in *Health Affairs* in 2007. In *Lancet Oncology* in that same year, Arduino Verdecchia published data demonstrating that American cancer patients have survival rates for all major cancers better than those in Western Europe and far better than in the United Kingdom.

It seems the Commonwealth Fund rankings reflect subjective surveys about "perceptions and experiences of patients and physicians" more than statistical analysis. But just to be fair, let's look closer at the top-rated NHS system in Great Britain.

Great Britain's NHS

Britain's NHS was founded in 1948. Aneurin Bevan, father of the NHS declared that *"everyone should be treated alike in the matter of medical care."* The Beveridge Report, the blueprint for the NHS, promised *"a health service providing full preventive and curative treatment of every kind for every citizen without exceptions."*

In a review of single-payer healthcare systems around the world, authors John C. Goodman, Gerald L. Musgrave, and Devon M. Herrick explain the goal of NHS founders was to eliminate inequalities in health care based on age, sex, occupation, geographical location and – most importantly – income and social class. As Bevan stated it, *"the essence of a satisfactory health service is that rich and poor are treated alike, that poverty is not a disability and wealth is not advantaged."*

These lofty goals have been repeated in one form or another by many politicians in many countries. Just how well has Great Britain's NHS accomplished their goals?

They certainly have put enough money into the system. It provides free health care for all citizens of Great Britain. NHS receives about 160 Billion British pounds a year from the Department of Health to run England's healthcare system. That's roughly one-sixth of all government spending and nearly triple Britain's defense budget. The NHS is a vast bureaucracy boasting 1.7 million workers, the fifth-largest employer on the planet, according to the BBC.

Although there have been numerous reorganizations and reforms over the six plus decades since it was founded, no prime minister – not even Margaret Thatcher – has found the political will to make fundamental changes. Nigel Lawson, Chancellor of the Exchequer under Thatcher, famously said, *"The NHS is the closest thing the English have to a religion."*

British NHS Reality

The NHS reported in September 2014 that its hospital waiting lists soared to their highest point since 2006, with 3.2 million patients waiting for treatment *after diagnosis.* According to a June report by NHS England, more than 15% of patients referred by their general practitioner for "urgent" treatment after being diagnosed with suspected cancer waited more than 62 days to begin their first definitive treatment.

Although the NHS was intended to reduce the number of people seeking treatment at hospital emergency rooms, the number of ER visits is rising. Some patients actually visit the ER up to four times a week. The BBC reports *"nearly 12,000 people made more than 10 visits to the same unit in 2012-2013."* These figures can be directly attributed to problems in *access* to care.

In the 1980s, an official task force called the Black Report found little evidence that access to health care was any more equal than when the NHS was started. This despite the assurances from British ministers of health that they were leaving no stone unturned in a relentless quest to eliminate inequalities in healthcare. A follow-up second task force twenty years later, called the Acheson Report, found evidence that access had become less equal in the years between the two studies.

The problem of poor access to healthcare is so well known in Britain that the press refers to the NHS as a "postcode lottery". This refers to a person's chances for timely, high-quality treatment depends on the neighborhood or "postcode" in which he or she lives. *The Guardian* sums up the situation with this statement, *"Generally speaking, the poorer you are and the more socially deprived your area, the worse your care and access is likely to be."*

Some studies bear out this impression:

- Nonelderly Britons living in areas with the worst-performing hospitals were 42 percent more likely to die on any given day than the average for Britain as a whole.
- The nonelderly population living in regions with the best-performing hospitals were 24 percent less likely to die than the average for Britain as a whole.
- Overall, the study found that if health care inequity were merely decreased to 1983 levels, some 7,500 premature deaths among people younger than sixty-five could be avoided each year.
- One study found that if the proportion of cancer-related illnesses and deaths were the same in Britain's lowest socioeconomic groups as in the most affluent, there would be 16,600 fewer deaths from cancer each year.
- The British Heart Foundation (BHF) found that the premature death rate for working-class men is 58 percent higher than non-working class men; the BHF estimates that more than 5,000 working-class men under the age of sixty-five die of coronary heart disease each year in Britain because of variations in health care *access* for different socioeconomic groups.

On a personal note, I was traveling this summer in Europe and had dinner several nights with two couples from England. One of the men had a total knee replacement recently and had to wait ten months for the surgery after diagnosis. He said the wait would have been much longer but he got special treatment because the surgeon had a close relationship with his rugby team. The usual wait can be up to two years.

This preferential treatment for those with the right connections is exactly what the founders of the NHS were determined to prevent. But the goals of those founders have long been dismissed as the public seeks to find ways to survive in a system that is clearly broken.

Dr. Mark Porter, Chairman of the council at the British Medical Association, has been quoted describing NHS's problems this way: *"A growing and aging population, public health problems like obesity, and constant advances in treatment and technology are all contributing to push NHS costs well above general inflation."*

Cal Thomas, syndicated columnist for *The Washington Examiner*, says many in Britain are beginning to question whether the country should continue its National Health Service. He warns that the United States could learn something from Britain's experience with a nationalized health system.

He writes that even the liberal British media is throwing in the towel on the NHS. Judith Woods, columnist for the *Daily Telegraph* says, *"It's time to make difficult decisions about the NHS. The NHS, dying on its feet for decades, is in a critical state. The promised injection of cash may stabilize it temporarily, but the chances of a full recovery are nil."* A headline in *The Guardian* declares the NHS is *"on the brink of extinction."*

Thomas also writes of a disturbing trend. In Britain, the National Institute for Health and Care Excellence (NICE) is the guiding body that determines what treatments are available and for whom. They decide whether new medicines should be approved. In 2005 they advised that smokers and obese people should be refused health care. As a result NHS North Yorkshire and York are preventing certain operations for the obese and smokers because they say unhealthy lifestyles lower their chance of success, according to the Heartland Institute.

NICE is the British equivalent of the Independent Payment Advisory Board (IPAB) created by ObamaCare. Although not yet operational, it will have similar authority to influence the course of medical treatment in America's future. Critics of ObamaCare were chastised for talk of "death panels" but the NHS is already demonstrating how government panels are influencing the treatments available to those in Great Britain.

The Canadian Experience

What about our neighbors to the north? Many supporters of ObamaCare look to Canada with envy believing their single-payer system is better than American healthcare. They say Canadians receive "free" healthcare and the quality is as good as we enjoy in America.

But Canadians don't agree. Bacchus Barua, health economist, and Jason Clemens, executive vice-president with the Fraser Institute make it clear that health care in Canada is anything but free. The average Canadian family of four pays approximately $11,320 in taxes for hospital and physician care through the country's tax system. This makes it the second most expensive health care system in the Organization for Economic Co-operation and Development (OECD) comprised of 14 countries.

Like most socialized medicine countries, Canada has a severe problem with *access* to health care. In 2013 the average wait time for an MRI was over two months; for a CT scan it was almost a month. In the same year, Canadians, on average, faced a four and a half months wait for medically necessary treatment *after* referral by a general practitioner. Furthermore, the problem is getting worse since this wait time is almost twice as long as it was in 1993 when it was first measured.

A study released in 2014 calculated some of the cost of these waiting times. The Fraser Institute found Canada's growing wait times for health care may have contributed to the deaths of 44,273 Canadian women between 1993 and 2009. The Fraser Institute is an independent, non-partisan Canadian public policy think-tank.

They calculated that for every one-week increase in the post-referral wait time for medically necessary elective procedures, three female Canadians died (per 100,000 women).

Study author Nadeem Esmail could not account for the gender differences in the study, which found no such relationship between wait times and male mortality. Possible factors include an increased participation among women in the workforce and differences in access to medical services. The author summarized the need for reform thus:

"Countries with relatively short health care wait times rely to varying degrees on market incentives and private competition, such as cost-sharing and competing private hospitals, within the universal health care system. Policymakers who cling to flawed policies, and argue against reform with rhetoric rather than fact, should consider whether Canadians who die while waiting for health care are being sacrificed to ideology."

Another Canadian, Dr. David Gratzer, writes of his own Canadian experiences. Born and raised in Canada he confesses to once believing that government health care is compassionate and equitable. Now he believe it is neither.

He says his views changed in medical school when he began to see how the system really worked; or didn't work. The problems were especially brought home when a relative had difficulty walking and had chronic pain. His doctor suggested a referral to a neurologist; an MRI was also needed and perhaps referral to another specialist. The expected wait time was roughly a year. Then, if surgery were recommended, there would be many months more waiting. Instead, he had the surgery done at the Mayo Clinic in the U.S. where he paid for it himself.

In fact, he says, Canadian medicine relies on American medicine. Between 2006 and 2008, Ontario sent more than 160 patients to New York and Michigan for emergency neurosurgery – described by the *Globe and Mail* newspaper as "broken necks, burst aneurysms, and other types of bleeding in or around the brain."

Waiting times in emergency rooms achieve national and international standards only half the time according to a government study. The physicians to population ratios are one of the lowest in the developed world, compounding the problem of access to health care. As a result, the physician shortage is so severe that some towns hold lotteries with the winners gaining access to the local doctor.

According to a study published in *Lancet Oncology* in 2013, five-year cancer survival rates are higher in the U.S. than in Canada. Based on data from the Joint Canada/U.S. Survey of Health, Americans have greater access to preventive screening tests and have higher treatment rates for chronic illnesses. Gratzer responds to these figures thus:

"No wonder: To limit the growth in health spending, governments restrict the supply of health care by rationing it through waiting. The same survey data show, as June and Paul O'Neill note in a paper published in 2007 in the Forum for Health Economics & Policy, that the poor under socialized medicine seem to be less healthy relative to the non-poor than their American counterparts."

He finds it ironic that the U.S. is on the verge of rushing toward government health care while Canada is reforming its system in the opposite direction. In 2005, Canada's Supreme Court struck down key laws in Quebec that established a government monopoly of health services. Claude Castonguay, who headed the Quebec government commission that recommended the creation of its public healthcare system in the 1960s, confessed to second thoughts. Last year, after completing another review, he declared the system in "crisis" and suggested a massive expansion of private services – even advocating that public hospitals rent facilities to physicians in off-hours.

Madam Chief Justice Beverley McLachlin of the Canadian Supreme Court wrote in that 2005 ruling that struck down the ban on private health insurance, *"Access to a waiting list is not access to health care."*

Private Sector Growing

The result is the growth of private health care in Canada – at a time when the Obama administration is trying to stifle private health care. Dr. Brian Day, an orthopedic surgeon, built a private hospital in Vancouver in the 1990s. Last year, he completed a term as the President of the Canadian Medical Association and was succeeded by a Quebec radiologist who owns several private clinics.

Dr. Day says the private sector of health care is growing in Canada. He estimates that 50,000 people are seen at private clinics every year in British Columbia. According to *The New York Times*, a private clinic opens at a rate of about one a week across the country.

The private sector is growing in Canada because the public sector is failing. Despite the fact that in 1999, Health Minister Allan Rock declared, *"Equal access regardless of financial means will continue to be a cornerstone of our system"*, there is little evidence this goal was ever achieved. Studies by The University of British Columbia consistently found wide-spread inequality in the provision of care among British Columbia's twenty or so health regions.

A comparison of two regions is illuminating. The study compares residents of Vancouver, population of almost two million, and Peace River, a rural area with a population of about 60,000.

- Residents of Vancouver received almost three times more specialist services per person than residents of Peace River, and this inequality held for groups with comparable health needs, males and females, and across all age groups..
- The differences were even more striking for certain specialties, with a five-to-one difference in the services of

internists and a thirty-one-to-one difference in the services of psychiatrists.

- Vancouver residents also enjoyed about 60 percent more General Practitioner services
- Spending on specialist services in Vancouver was almost four times higher than spending on specialists in rural Cariboo.
- Per capita spending on all services was almost three times as high in Vancouver ($609) as in Peace River ($231).

Barua and Clemens summarize the Canadian healthcare system with these ominous words:

"The reality of Canadian health care is that it is comparatively expensive and imposes enormous costs on Canadians in the form of waiting for services, and limited access to physicians and medical technology. This isn't something any country should consider replicating".

The Swedish Experience

What about Sweden? They were ranked 3rd by the Commonwealth Fund. Many people tout Sweden as the best example of a socialized system that works. But what do the Swedish people say?

Per Bylund, Swedish economist and professor at Baylor University's Hankamer School of Business, tells a different story. Writing in *The Wall Street Journal,* Bylund says the overall quality of medical services delivered by Sweden's universal public health care is consistently among the world's best.

But the problem again is *access* to care. According to the Euro Health Consumer Index 2013, Swedish patients suffer from inordinately long waiting times to get an appointment with a doctor, specialist treatment, or even emergency care.

He gives examples. Sweden's National Board of Health and Welfare reports that as of 2013, the average wait time from referral to start of treatment for "intermediary and high risk" prostate cancer is an incredible 220 days. In the case of lung cancer, which is much more deadly, the wait between an appointment with a specialist and a treatment decision is 37 days.

One 80 year-old Swedish woman recently had to wait four hours before an ambulance arrived. And no ambulance at all came to a one-month-old infant who suffered a cerebral hemorrhage.

A 42 year-old woman in Karlstad seeking care for meningitis died in the ER after a three-hour wait. A woman with colon cancer spent 12 years contesting a money-saving decision to deny an abdominal scan that would have found the cancer earlier. The denial-of-care decision was not made by an insurance company, but by the government healthcare system and its policies.

Rationing of Healthcare

In Great Britain, Canada, and Sweden (and our own VA system) there is a problem with *access* to care. The people get free coverage of their healthcare – *when they can get it!* Economists call this *rationing* – the delay or even failure to provide care due to government budgetary decisions. Expect the same in this country soon with ObamaCare.

We will experience the same problems of rationing of healthcare because ObamaCare increases the number of people with health insurance without increasing the supply of healthcare providers, nor increasing their incentives to provide that care. There are no provisions in ObamaCare to increase the number of doctors at a time when we already have a doctor shortage.

In fact, the onerous provisions of ObamaCare have led about 40% of the existing doctors to plan early retirement or a change in professions to non-clinical care. This number shows up repeatedly on surveys of doctors. The result will be a much greater doctor shortage than we already have. Combine this with an increased volume of patients demanding healthcare (due to increased numbers with government subsidized health insurance or Medicaid) and you have a big *access to healthcare* problem. The only way to deal with this problem is *rationing* of care by delays in treatment.

The Move to Privatization

Ironically, at a time when America is moving more toward socialized medicine, Great Britain, Canada, and Sweden are moving away from it; at least in practical if not ideological ways. All three countries are looking to private medicine to provide for the backlog of treatment the public medicine can't handle.

In Sweden, Insurance Sweden, the country's national insurance company trade organization, reports that in 2013 12% of working adults had private insurance even though they are already "guaranteed" public healthcare. The number of private policy holders has increased by 67% over the last five years, despite the fact that an average Swedish family already pays nearly $20,000 annually in taxes toward healthcare and elderly care. Almost 600,000 Swedes now use private insurance even though public healthcare is free.

Ten years ago, the Swedish government approved the corporate management of St. Goran Hospital in Stockholm by Capio, a private corporation owned by venture capitalists based in London and Stockholm. The hospital provides health care services to the Swedish people paid for with Swedish taxpayer's money.

Randeep Ramesh, writing for *The Guardian*, a British newspaper, says the British government of Prime Minister David Cameron is considering such a future for the National Health Service of Great Britain. This privatization of health care is a product of a coalition of liberals and conservatives in Sweden that has brought in for-profit free schools in education, sliced welfare to pay off the deficit and has privatized large parts of the health service.

There are now six private hospitals funded by the Swedish taxpayers, comprising about 8 percent of the total.

In an interview with Ramesh, St. Goran's chief executive, Britt Wallgren, said the 310-bed hospital, which serves 430,000 people, outperforms state-owned rivals inside and outside the country. She says emergency patients see a doctor within half an hour compared with up to four hours for patients waiting in Britain's NHS hospitals.

Capio president Thomas Berglund says the *"profit motive works in healthcare"* and companies run on *"capitalism, not altruism."*

Similar moves toward privatization are happening in Canada as we already discussed.

In Great Britain, about six million British citizens buy private health insurance and about 250,000 choose to pay for private treatment out-of-pocket each year – though NHS insurance costs $3,500 annually for every British man, woman, and child. The backlog for NHS treatment is so long that NHS actually funds some private treatment.

The share of NHS-funded hip and knee replacements by private doctors increased to 19% in 2011-12, from a negligible amount in 2003-2004. If the Cameron government indeed is envious of the privatization moves in Sweden, it is likely the NHS will be funding more private health care in the future.

Is Switzerland Better?

The Swiss are often given credit for one of the most egalitarian health care systems in the world. Although there are some portions of the Swiss system worth considering, there is more to consider with caution. John C. Goodman of *The National Center for Policy Analysis* wrote the following assessment of the Swiss:

"Here's the good, the bad, and the ugly:

- **The Good** – *Swiss health care is predominantly private. Individuals are required to buy insurance and almost all of them do. Private companies compete to provide insurance, and there are subsidies for lower income buyers. The insurance is individually owned, personal and portable. In my opinion, this system stands head and shoulders above other European systems of national health insurance.*
- **The Bad** – *Despite competition, choice, private ownership and portability, the Swiss system is still very bureaucratic – perhaps*

as much as or more so than our own. It has mandated benefits, price controls on providers and other regulations that make it hard for entrepreneurs to solve problems in the way we often talk about here.

- ***The Ugly** – Although long-term insurance relationships are the norm, the Swiss have been moving in the direction of managed competition, which encourages people to switch health plans. As I have written before, when plans are forced to charge community-rated premiums, no one ever faces a real price, pays a real price, or receives a real price. Under managed competition, everyone's incentives are perverse."*

Goodman explains that with managed competition, on the buyer side, people have an incentive to underinsure when they are healthy and overinsure when they are sick. On the seller side, health plans have an incentive to overprovide to the healthy (on whom they make a profit) and underprovide to the sick (on whom they incur losses). The more competitive the market, the worse these perverse outcomes will be.

Avik Roy, writing in *The Weekly Standard,* points out that countries like Switzerland and Singapore, on the other hand, have the lowest per-capita public health spending in the world. Switzerland spends $1,628 per person and Singapore spends $813 per person (Figure 1). How do they keep their costs low? Roy gives three reasons:

- Both countries use the power of private markets
- Switzerland has no government-run insurers, though 20 percent of its population receives government premium subsidies.
- Singapore uses health savings accounts and high-deductible insurance plans to keep costs low.

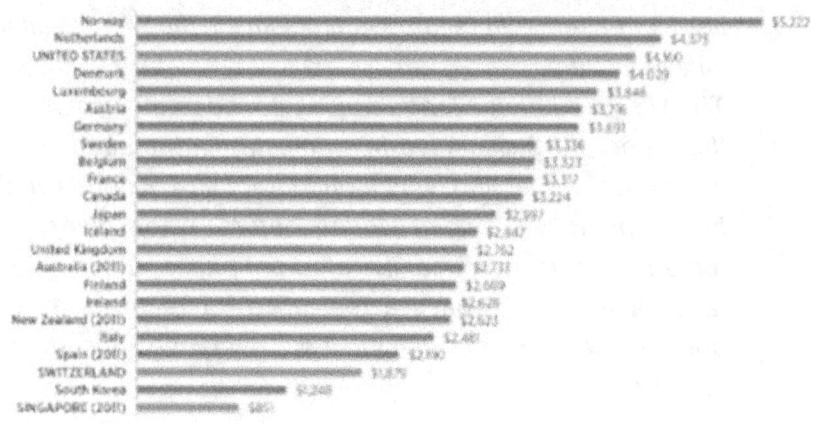

Figure 1 – 2012 Public Health Expenditures per Capita by country.

Efficiency Measures

How do countries compare on their efficiency in providing health care? How much does it cost a hospital to perform an appendectomy? Goodman says outside the United States, it is doubtful that any public hospital could provide the answer. Nor do government-run hospitals typically keep records that would allow anyone else to find out.

Health economist Alain Enthoven has observed that because health care in Britain is so politicized, "*It is more difficult to close an unneeded British hospital than an unneeded American military base.*"

Great Britain has about 20 percent fewer inpatient hospital beds per capita than the United States and about 44 percent fewer than the OCED median of 4.3 per 1,000 population. As a result, bed shortages are common. What's worse, Britain also has staffing shortages making it impossible to utilize all of the beds they have.

More than one million people are waiting for medical treatment in British hospitals at any one time and an estimated 500,000 surgeries were cancelled in the past five years due to the shortage of NHS hospital beds. Yet close to 30,000 beds (16 percent of the total) are empty on any given day. Add to that the number of beds filled with patients who do not belong in a hospital at all and this implies that one out of every three NHS hospital beds are unavailable for acute care patients.

In Canada, a large percentage of acute care hospital beds also are used for patients who do not need acute care. The Manitoba Center for Health Policy found that across the provinces from 7 percent to 51 percent of Canadian adult admissions and from 27 percent to 59 percent of the days patients spend in hospitals were for conditions that did not require acute care, although most did need some form of supervised care.

- In Manitoba, 23 percent of the bed days spent by short-stay patients in acute care hospitals were unnecessary.
- In Winnipeg, Manitoba, 40 percent of the acute care beds were used by only a few patients, each staying more than thirty days.

One of the most widely used measures of hospital efficiency is average length of stay (LOS). The inappropriate use of hospital facilities has a significant impact on the efficiency of the health care system. The lower the LOS, the more efficient the system. By this standard, the United States hospitals are ahead of their international counterparts:

- **United States – average LOS – 5.9 days**
- United Kingdom – average LOS – 6.2 days
- Australia – average LOS – 6.2 days
- Germany – average LOS – 9.6 days
- Canada – average LOS – 7.1 days
- OECD Median – average LOS – 6.4 days

This is consistent with my own career observations. When I began my medical school training in the 1970s, patients spent much more time in the hospital for even minor operations. Procedures like arthroscopic knee surgery usually consisted of admission the day before surgery followed by three more days after surgery. Today this same procedure is routinely done as an outpatient with no hospital stay at all. American doctors are always looking for ways to do treatment without the need for hospitalization. Doctors and patients prefer it that way and studies show patients suffer fewer complications when they are not in the hospital.

Cost Comparisons

A study was done comparing the costs for providing health care in the British NHS to Kaiser Permanente, a large U.S. HMO. The study concluded that the per capita costs of the two systems were similar. However, the analysis found Kaiser provided its member with more comprehensive and convenient primary care services and much more rapid access to specialists and hospital admissions.

The comparison showed the NHS costs were calculated at $1,764 per capita compared to Kaiser costs of $1,951 per capita. However, there were significant differences noted:

- Kaiser had two and one-half times as many pediatricians, twice as many obstetricians-gynecologists and three times as many cardiologists per enrollee as the NHS.
- After referral, waiting times to see a specialist were more than six times as long in the NHS.
- For nonemergency hospital admission, 90 percent of Kaiser patients waited less than three months; one-third of NHS patients waited more than five months.
- Kaiser had 270 acute care bed days /1000 population, whereas NHS patients stayed three times longer – an average of 1000 acute care days/1000 population.

The study concluded the following: *"The widely held beliefs that the NHS is efficient and that poor performance in certain areas is largely explained by underinvestment are not supported by this analysis. Kaiser achieved better performance at roughly the same cost as the NHS because of integration throughout the system, efficient management of hospital use, the benefits of competition and greater investment in information technology."*

Avoiding Rationing

There is a common theme running through all of these socialized medicine countries – long waiting times to receive health care treatment. In a socialized model, the only way to slow the growth of health care spending is by denying services - *rationing* - not by using medical resources more efficiently.

Under the old Soviet Union, the people had to wait in lines, sometimes for days, to buy bread and other basic foodstuffs because the government didn't want to spend any more money. The same happens with health care when government healthcare budgets cannot keep pace with demand.

Per Bylund sums up the situation well: *"It is possible to have truly affordable, qualitative and accessible care. But the only way to get this result is through a system where providers freely compete with each other to lower costs and raise quality. There is no short cut to well-functioning, affordable health care. Sweden's undesirable experience shows this very clearly."*

The answer is not socialized medicine. We'll discuss in the next chapter the recent VA system scandals that illustrate what socialized medicine leads to - people dying while they wait to receive healthcare. The answer is a competitive system of private health care that incentivizes doctors to provide more care at lower cost and higher quality and gives patients the freedom to choose their own doctor and their own treatment.

7

The VA Scandal

"The Administration and Congress have failed to ensure our nation is living up to the promises we have made to our veterans."
Senator Tom Coburn (R - OK) - 6/24/14

Socialized medicine is already here. Socialized medicine has existed in this country since before the establishment of the Republic. We need only look at the healthcare provided to our military veterans to see how well socialized medicine really works.

History of the VA
In 1636, the Pilgrims of Plymouth Colony were at war with the Pequot Indians. The Pilgrims passed a law, which stated that disabled soldiers would be supported by the colony.

The Continental Congress of 1776 recognized the need for support of the military if they were to be able to recruit a sufficient military to fight the war for independence. They provided pensions for soldiers who were disabled. Direct medical and hospital care was given to veterans in the early days of the Republic and was provided by the individual States and communities.

In 1811, the first domiciliary and medical facility for veterans was authorized by the Federal Government. Later in the 19th century, the Nation's veterans assistance program was expanded to increase benefits and pensions not only for veterans but also their widows and dependents.

After the Civil War, many State-run veterans homes were established. Since domiciliary care was available at all State veterans homes, incidental medical and hospital treatment was provided for all injuries and diseases, whether service connected or not. Indigent and disabled veterans of the Civil war, Indian Wars, Spanish-American War, and Mexican Border period as well as discharged regular members of the Armed Forces were cared for at these homes.

World War I brought new changes to the system. Congress established a new system of veterans' benefits when the United States entered the war in 1917. These new benefits included programs for disability compensation, insurance for service persons and veterans, and vocational rehabilitation for the disabled. By the 1920s, the benefits were administered by three different Federal agencies: the Veterans Bureau, the Bureau of Pensions of the Interior Department, and the National Home for Disabled Volunteer Soldiers.

The Veterans Administration that we know today was established by Congress in 1930. It authorized the President to "consolidate and coordinate government activities affecting war veterans." The three component agencies became bureaus within the Veterans Administration. Brigadier General Frank T. Hines, who directed the Veterans Bureau for seven years, was named as the first Administrator of Veterans Affairs, a job he held from 1930 to 1945.

The modern VA is a product of the vast number of veterans returning from the battles of World War II needing medical services. The combination of four million elderly veterans from World War I, and fifteen million returning soldiers from World War II, required a vast expansion of veterans' health care. There were not yet established entitlements like Medicaid and Medicare and there were far fewer hospitals than exist today.

Since that time the VA health care system has grown from 54 hospitals in 1930 to 152 hospitals, 800 community-based outpatient clinics, 126 nursing home care units, and 35 domiciliaries. VA health care facilities provide a broad spectrum of medical, surgical, and rehabilitative care, serving 5.7 million patients.

World War II resulted in not only a vast increase in the veteran population, but also in large numbers of new benefits enacted by the Congress for veterans of the war. The GI Bill, signed into law June 22, 1944, is said to have had more impact on the American way of life than any law since the Homestead Act of 1862. It provided educational assistance for every military veteran and enabled millions to begin new careers after the war.

The Department of Veterans Affairs (VA) was established as a Cabinet-level position on March 15, 1989, by President George H.W. Bush. President Bush, a World War II naval pilot and war hero, elevated the role of the VA saying,

"There is only one place for the veterans of America, in the Cabinet Room, at the table with the President of the United States of America."

In 2013, the VA spent $56 billion on medical care, up from $40 billion in 2009 and $19 billion in 1998. With over 300,000 employees, the VA is the second-largest department of the federal government.

Socialized Medicine

The term "socialized medicine" is used widely to describe health care systems administered by the federal government. But there are actually several different models of such systems that vary in terms of the ownership of the facilities and the employers of the providers. Avik Roy, healthcare blogger for *Forbes,* designates at least three such systems in common usage:

Socialized Medicine – properly understood, is a system in which the state owns and controls everything. The government owns the hospitals; it employs the physicians; it pays for the health insurance and the health care. That, in a nutshell, is the **VA.** It's also, for the most part, the system in place under the **British National Health Service (NHS).**

Single-payer Health Care – is only partly socialized. In a single-payer system, the government is the sole insurer, but hospitals can be widely privately owned and operated, and doctors can work for private hospitals or for themselves. **Medicare** and **Medicaid**, at the outset, were designed as single payer programs. **Canada** has such a system for their health care.

Subsidized Private Health Care – is the next step downward, in terms of government intervention. In countries like **Switzerland**, for example, there are no government insurers or "public options." Instead, the Swiss government offers premium support subsidies for low-income individuals to shop for private insurance. Under this model, the government often regulates the types of insurance products that are eligible for subsidies.

Which system is best? Switzerland is renowned for its high patient satisfaction, low wait times, and access to the latest technology. But it is far from perfect with the government restricting what types of procedures are permissible and what insurance policies must include. Medicaid provides poor quality coverage and access to care is very limited since many doctors refuse to accept Medicaid patients. Medicare is slightly better but is heading down the same path as Medicaid. Private medicine in America is expensive, but generally considered to have high quality, in many instances the best in the world.

ObamaCare borrows from each of these systems in expanding coverage for Americans. First, it takes from the Swiss-style exchanges to provide subsidized, regulated private insurance plans. Second, it expands Medicaid. Third, it allows the continuation of private insurance – but regulates closely the type of insurance available and mandates everyone purchase it. It raises the cost of this insurance by insisting upon the coverage of pre-existing medical conditions and by using "community rating" for determination of premiums, which raises the cost for patients and insurers alike.

The expansion of insurance coverage through government-run insurance exchanges may improve the quality of healthcare for some individuals. But the quality will certainly not approach that of private insurance since the exchanges only offer narrow networks without the leading physicians and hospitals.

The expansion of Medicaid will certainly not improve health outcomes relative to the uninsured as we discussed in Chapter Four. Unfortunately, Medicare will soon find itself in the same situation since federal funding of the program has been slashed $716 billion over the next decade to pay for ObamaCare. Medicare actuaries predict Medicare fees to providers will be less than Medicaid by the year 2020. When that happens, Medicare patients will find themselves in the same difficult situation trying to get health care as Medicaid patients are in today.

The VA System

That brings us to the VA. As noted above, the VA system is a true socialized medicine model; all hospitals, clinics, and other facilities, as well as all doctors and medical staff, are employees of the government. The government pays all the bills, makes all the rules, controls all the decision-making, and hires all the medical providers. As a result, they provide the worst healthcare system in America.

This has long been the opinion of most who have ever worked in the VA system. Roy continues his observations:

"Anyone who has ever worked at a VA hospital can tell you what a terrible experience it can be. Yale-New Haven Hospital, where I did many of my clinical rotations, is far from perfect – but heading out to the West Haven VA was like traversing the Iron Curtain. The problems facing the VA system will be familiar to anyone who has dealt with the British NHS: unsanitary conditions, leading to higher rates of hospital-borne infections; rationing of drugs and procedures, leading to poorer health outcomes; and on and on."

Hal Scherz, a pediatric urological surgeon in private practice who also serves on the faculty of Emory University Medical School, wrote of his own experiences in a *Wall Street Journal* Op-ed. Scherz writes:

"Most doctors have their personal VA stories. In my experience at VA hospitals in San Antonio and San Diego, patients were seen in clinics that were understaffed and overscheduled. Appointments for X-rays and other tests had to be scheduled months in advance,

and longer for surgery. Hospital administrators limited operating time, making sure that work stopped by 3 p.m. Consequently, the physician in charge kept a list of patients who needed surgery and rationed the available slots to those with the most urgent problems.

Scott Barbour, an orthopedic surgeon and a friend, trained at the Miami VA hospital. In an attempt to get more patients onto the operating-room schedule, he enlisted fellow residents to clean the operating rooms between cases and transport patients from their rooms into the surgical suites. Instead of offering praise for their industriousness, the chief of surgery reprimanded the doctors and put a stop to their actions. From his perspective, they were not solving a problem but were making federal workers look bad, and creating more work for others, like nurses, who had to take care of more post-op patients.

At the VA hospital in St. Louis, urologist Michael Packer, a former partner of mine, had difficulty getting charts from the medical records department. He and another resident hunted them down themselves. It was easier for department workers to say that they couldn't find a chart than to go through the trouble of looking. Without these records, patients could not receive care, which was an unacceptable situation to these doctors. Not long after they began doing this, they were warned to stand down.

In my experience, the best thing that a patient in the VA system could hope for was that the services he needed were unavailable. When that is the case, the VA outsources their care to doctors in the community, where their problems are promptly addressed. But these patients still need to return to the VA system for other services and get back on a long waiting list."

My own experience in medical training concurs with these observations. Nearly every physician ever trained in this country spends time in a local VA hospital as a part of the required rotations of clinical experience. My exposure to this system happened at the Philadelphia VA Hospital in the 1970s.

Nowhere have I experienced greater bureaucratic interference with the delivery of health care. Since there is no competition to the VA system there is no incentive for delivery of better care. Accountability for VA staff is lacking and union protections and regulations make firing incompetent workers nearly impossible.

I was immediately struck by the callous attitude of hospital staff who had learned long ago that they had little chance of being fired for lack of performance. Ward clerks spent their days doing as little as possible to get by, leaving the work to medical students and residents to pick up the pieces. Nurses seemed unmotivated to do more than necessary to make patients comfortable. Even hospital medical staff showed no inclination to perform more than a rudimentary number of elective procedures since as salaried workers they had no incentive to do more.

The system fails because there is no accountability and no incentives to do better or accomplish more. In fact, those that would seek to improve are generally criticized by co-workers for "making us look bad." Such attitudes sow the seeds for failure.

The VA Scandal

By this time nearly everyone in America knows there is a scandal involving the Veterans Affairs Hospitals that provide healthcare to our military veterans. The debate now is what to do about it, whom to hold accountable, and determining the implications of this complete failure of the VA system for the future of ObamaCare.

For those of you unfamiliar with this story, let me briefly review the known facts. According to the Inspector General report, the reports of fraudulent documentation of waiting times for veterans to receive medical treatment at the Phoenix VA Hospital are worse than initial claims. The IG report found primary-care waiting times averaged 115 days, nearly five times what the hospital reported and eight times the VA's 14 day target. About 3100 veterans were actually waiting in line and more than half of them weren't on the official waiting list.

Whistleblowers at the hospital allege that forty or more veterans died while waiting to receive treatment.

This problem is not unique to the Phoenix VA Hospital alone. At this time 42 VA medical centers are under investigation for similar problems. This is not actually a new problem. According to an editorial in *The Wall Street Journal*, this is the 19th IG report since 2005 to document excessive wait times at VA Hospitals.

It is not the intent of this author to place blame on the Obama administration alone for these failures. The problems at the VA have existed for years, through both Republican and Democratic administrations. It is true that President Obama was briefed on this exact problem when he first took the office of the presidency in 2009 and there is little evidence he has done much about it except increase the VA budget. This common liberal solution to any problem has failed miserably. But that's precisely the point. More money is not the solution. The problems are more endemic to the nature of the institution.

Dr. Sam Foote is an internist who worked for the VA system in Phoenix for 23 years. In recent years he became concerned when he saw that too many veterans were not receiving the care they needed. He wrote letters to the VA Office of the Inspector General charging that Phoenix-area veterans had died waiting months for care, hidden on secret waiting lists. Then he reached out to the media. Soon, other whistleblowers acknowledged the same problems at other VA hospitals.

The subsequent investigation revealed 57,000 veterans had been waiting more than three months for an initial appointment and another 64,000 veterans had requested an appointment over the past decade but weren't even on the waiting list. These people had either fallen through the cracks of the system or had been kept on secret lists designed to make the facilities appear more efficient than they were.

What provoked this situation? In the 1990s, with the population of WW II veterans shrinking, the VA opened eligibility for health care to more veterans. Between 1997 and 2001, the number of veterans using VA health care services jumped 40 percent, to 3.7 million. The wars in Afghanistan and Iraq only added to those numbers.

Then the economy declined in 2008. This increased the stress on VA resources since many veterans lost their private health insurance and began using the VA as a backup system. *"Whenever the economy tanks, more people come to the VA,"* Foote says. *"People would come in and say, 'This is the first time I've used my benefits because I was on my wife's insurance' or 'I had my own insurance and I lost my job.'"*

Between 2002 and 2012, the number of VA health care enrollees increased nationwide by a third to 9 million. Outpatient visits to VA facilities nearly doubled to 83 million per year. In the last three years alone, primary care visits increased 50 percent, but the number of primary care providers grew only by 9 percent. Naturally, the result was even longer waiting times.

Foote tells of a meeting in 2012 to discuss strategies for handling the crisis of increasing demand for services. He recalls the only answer discussed: *"But they came up with one: Fake the numbers. Simple. That was the solution."*

The problem of long waiting times was nothing new to the Inspector General. He had issued 18 reports since 2005 documenting delays in care nationwide. In 2011 the VA had set a goal that patients should be seen within 14 days of requesting an appointment. Knowing they could not meet this expectation, Phoenix VA, and many other facilities, found ways to fudge the numbers.

For instance, if a veteran requested an appointment but the first available slot was five months away, the system handled the situation as Foot explains: If the veteran agreed to that time – even though he wanted care much sooner – a VA scheduler could mark the wait time as zero days.

But wait, it gets much worse! Foote says, *"No one was allowed to make new patient appointments in the computer."* Instead, appointment requests were kept on separate, unofficial lists until an opening drew close, when they were moved onto the "official list", giving the illusion of efficiency and meeting their goal for an appointment within 14 days of request. Since there were financial rewards for meeting the goal, employees had good incentives to cook the books.

Foote mentions other tricks concocted to "game the system". *"Let's say you have 10 patients you see a day in your clinic. You want to have an easy day? Have your staff make appointments for people who are dead."* He also said doctors and staff would call a patient the night before an appointment, tell him he needed to bring additional paperwork, and reschedule his appointment for three weeks later.

Foote, with the help of a colleague, finally began gathering the names of patients waiting for care and turned them over to the inspector general. When scheduling clerks called these patients to make an appointment they learned that many had been waiting months for an appointment – and some had died.

Foote first began calling the situation to the attention of the inspector general in June 2013. It took six months for an investigation to begin but in December the IG sent a team to Phoenix. Foote heard little and wrote another letter of concern to the IG in March. When the results of their investigation were finally released, the news was worse than even Foote suspected. The IG team found 1,400 veterans had waited at least three months for a first appointment. Forty or more veterans had died awaiting care.

Since then other whistleblowers have come forward to share their own horror stories. Now we know the problem is not limited to Phoenix but is rampant throughout the whole VA system.

The Scandal Gets Worse

Just when the scandal seemed too bad to believe, it only got worse. A Senate investigation led by Senator Tom Coburn (R –OK) revealed far more dirt has been uncovered about the VA that shows the problems there go much deeper than falsified waiting times.

Senator Coburn released his new oversight report, *"Friendly Fire: Death, Delay, and Dismay at the VA."* This report is based on a year-long investigation of VA hospitals across the nation that documents inappropriate conduct and incompetence at the VA that led to well-documented deaths and delays. Furthermore, it reveals inept congressional and agency oversight that allowed these problems to grow unchecked.

Dr. Coburn, an obstetrician-gynecologist, explains: *"The Administration and Congress have failed to ensure our nation is living up to the promises we have made to our veterans. As a physician who has personally cared for hundreds of Oklahoma veterans, this is intolerable. As a senator, I'm determined to address the structural challenges of the Department of Veterans Affairs so we can end this national disgrace and improve quality and access to health care for our veterans."*

Findings of the Report

The key findings in the report include:

- The cover up of waiting lists for doctor's appointments at the VA is just the tip of the iceberg, reflecting a perverse culture within the department where veterans are not always the priority and data and employees are manipulated to maintain the appearance that all is well.
- Bad employees are rewarded with bonuses and paid leave while whistleblowers, healthcare providers, and even veterans and their families are subjected to bullying, sexual harassment, abuse, and neglect. For example, female patients received unnecessary pelvic and breast exams from a sex offender, a noose was left on the desk of a minority employee by a co-worker, and a nurse who murdered a veteran harassed the family of the deceased to get them to admit guilt for the death.
- The care at more centers is getting worse and some VA health care providers have lost their medical licenses, and the VA is hiding this information from patients.
- Delays exist for more than just doctors' appointments – disability claims, construction, urgent care, and registries are also slow or behind schedule.

- Despite a nursing shortage, many VA nurses spend their days conducting union activities to advocate for better conditions for themselves rather than veterans.

Tragic Consequences

The tragic consequences of this scandal of mismanagement are highlighted in the report:

- The report identifies $20 Billion in waste and mismanagement that could have been better spent providing health care to veterans.
- More than 1,000 veterans may have died as a result of VA misconduct over the past decade.
- The federal government has paid out $845 million for VA medical malpractice since 2001.
- Most VA construction projects are over budget and behind schedule, inflating costs by billions of dollars.

Who is responsible? There is plenty of blame to spread around for a problem that has existed for more than a decade under administrations of both parties. Yet the problems were well known when President Obama took office and he pledged to solve them. Unfortunately, there is little or no evidence that he did anything to provide the solution other than increasing the VA budget.

Senator Coburn's report identifies the following failures:

- The Senate Veterans Affairs Committee largely ignored the warnings about delays and dysfunction at the VA for decades, abdicating its oversight responsibilities and choosing to make new promises to veterans rather than making sure those promises already made were being kept.
- This report details how Congress was repeatedly alerted and warned of the problems plaguing the VA over decades.

- The Senate Veterans Affairs Committee has only held two oversight hearings the last four years, and was even profiled in *Wastebook 2012* for being among the committees in Congress holding the fewest number of hearings.

The Real Problem

What is the real problem behind these VA scandals? Mark Hemingway, writing in *The Weekly Standard* believes it is the inability of the government to hold incompetent VA employees accountable. He reports the VA has fired a grand total of three senior executives for performance failures in the last five years – one-fourth the federal average for terminations.

The Office of Personnel Management disclosed in 2013, only 0.47 percent of the federal workforce was terminated for cause, considerably below the 3.0 percent fired in the private sector. In 2011, USA Today reported that in at least 15 federal agencies, employees were more likely to die of natural causes than be terminated in any given year. Yet, the average federal employee made $126,141 in pay and benefits in 2012, more than double the private sector average.

Unions also contribute to the problem. Public employees' union dues flow into the unions' political contributions – which flow into Democratic coffers to maintain the status quo. Stopping this will require eliminating unions in government jobs. But even before this is achieved, we must stop union workers from being compensated by the taxpayer for union activities. In 2012, the IRS alone spent $21.6 million compensating employees who were working on union activities, not on public jobs. The Coburn report details how this same problem is widespread in the VA as well.

Kimberley Strassel, writing in *The Wall Street Journal,* details the impact of unions on the problem.

"The VA boast one of the largest federal workforces and VA Secretary Eric Shinseki bragged in 2010 that two-thirds of it is unionized. That's a whopping 200,000 union members, represented

by the likes of the American Federation of Government Employees and the Service Employees International Union. And this is government-run health care – something unions know a lot about from organizing health workers in the private sector. Compared with most D.C. unions the VA houses a serious union shop."

*"Manhattan Institute scholar Diana Furchtgott-Roth recently detailed Office of Personnel Management numbers obtained through a Freedom of Information Act request by Rep. Phil Gingrey (R- GA). On May 25, Ms. Furchtgott-Roth reported on MarketWatch that the VA in 2012 paid 258 employees to be 100% "full-time" receiving full pay and benefits to do **only** union work. Seventeen had six-figure salaries, up to $132,000. According to the Office of Personnel Management, the VA paid for 988,000 hours of 'official' time in fiscal 2011, a 23% increase from 2010."*

In other words, taxpayers are paying union workers to do union work, at the expense of the veterans they are supposed to be working for. Moreover, Strassel says the union is making the waiting-times problem even worse.

"As for patient-case backlogs, the unions have helped in their creation. Contract-negotiated work rules over job classifications and duties and seniorities are central to the 'bureaucracy' that fails veterans. More damaging has been the union hostility to any VA attempt to give veterans access to alternative sources of care – which the unions consider a direct job threat. The American Federation of Government Employees puts out regular press release blasting any 'out-sourcing' of VA work to non-VA- union members."

Solutions Proposed

The House of Representatives overwhelmingly passed bipartisan legislation, by a vote of 390-33, which would give the VA greater authority to fire or demote senior executives for performance. This additional firing flexibility would apply only to the top 360 supervisors out of more than 340,000 employees at the VA. Yet the bill was blocked in the Senate by Vermont's Bernie Sanders.

Instead, Sanders joined forces with Senator John McCain (R – AZ) to pass a different bill that would increase VA funding by $500 million to expedite hiring for new doctors, nurses and other staff. *The Wall Street Journal* reports this is on top of this year's $57.3 Billion VA budget, which is 106 % more than in 2003 though patients have increased by only 30 percent. The bill also gives the VA $236.9 million to lease or build 27 new major medical facilities in 18 states and Puerto Rico. And the Phoenix VA, first identified in this scandal for its dissembling and dysfunction resulting in preventable deaths, will be rewarded with a new $20.7 million "community-based outpatient clinic."

In typical Washington fashion, the solution proposed is to throw more money at the problem and hope something good happens. But increasing the VA budget, as President Obama already did, has done nothing to solve the problem, because the problems are entrenched within the system. Building more buildings and hiring more staff will never solve these problems.

The Senate legislation does make one good suggestion; issuing veterans a "choice card" to allow them to seek care outside the VA if the wait is longer than the two-week maximum. This partial privatization trial is scheduled to expire in two years. I would recommend this be made permanent so that veterans can be sure they will receive their care in a timely manner. Furthermore, this will hold VA executives accountable when they fail to meet their benchmarks.

Under bipartisan pressure, VA Secretary General Eric Shinseki was forced to resign. Although this may soothe some of the political wounds the Obama administration is nursing, it is unlikely to make a significant difference in the functioning of the VA Hospital system. While a better manager of the VA is surely needed, the problems of socialized medicine will remain.

The real solution is to privatize the system says Avik Roy, writing in *Forbes:*

"There is only one way to truly reform the VA, to truly ensure that veterans get the care they need. And that is to give vets the ability to

take the money that the government spends on them and use it to buy high-quality, private insurance. There are two straightforward ways to go about it. One would be to give veterans subsidies with which to buy insurance from the Federal Employee Health Benefits Program, the popular private health insurance program for government workers. Another would be to allow those same subsidies to be used on the ObamaCare insurance exchanges. Either approach would allow veterans to seek care from private hospitals and private physicians."

Considering that the ObamaCare exchanges offer only "narrow networks" shunned by the best doctors and hospitals, I would prefer our veterans be given option one. Dumping more people on the insurance exchanges will only exacerbate the waiting times those patients are likely to experience in the near future.

The *Wall Street Journal* editorialized their solution:

"Instead of paying for shorter delays, a better option is to fix the structure that causes delays. That means decentralizing the VA and selling off most of the institution. There is no medical or biological reason that former soldiers require special hospitals for routine treatments or even most complex conditions. The VA can prioritize specialized care for combat trauma and rehabilitation unique to military service, insurance vouchers for vets can replace socialized medicine, and markets will discipline a now-unaccountable bureaucratic culture."

Perhaps the most credible opinion on improving the VA situation comes from Kenneth W. Kizer, former Undersecretary of Veterans Affairs in charge of the VA health system under President Clinton from 1994 to 1999. Kizer modernized the VA's computer systems, fired poor-performing doctors, and established private-sector-style metrics to measure the VA's performance on patient wait times, according to Avik Roy, health care journalist for *Forbes*. The VA enjoyed a period of prosperity and improved performance under his leadership.

Writing in *The New England Journal of Medicine,* Kizer and coauthor Ashish K. Jha propose three steps to solving the current VA crisis:

- First – after ensuring all veterans on wait lists are screened and triaged for care, the VA should refocus its performance-management system on fewer measures that directly address what is most important to veteran patients and clinicians – *outcome measures.*
- Second – conceptualizing access to care in terms of a "continuous healing relationship," the agency should design a new access strategy that draws on modern information and *advanced communications technologies.*
- Third – engage more with *private-sector health care organizations* and the general public and make performance data broadly available. Transparency may expose vulnerabilities, but it is easier to improve when weaknesses are publicly acknowledged.

It is clear from the assessment of Kizer and Jha that just throwing more money at the problem is not the solution. *The Wall Street Journal* applauds their work and recommendations but offers a warning:

"After the Senate deal, look for the politicians in both parties to drop this issue and move on. The Kizer-Jha diagnosis is merely one among many showing that the VA's problems run far deeper than a new hospital building or more spending can solve, which means that the Senate's non-reform reform betrays veterans one more time."

VA Hospitals v. ObamaCare

What are the implications of this VA scandal for ObamaCare? Is there reason to believe we will see the same horror stories with the changes ObamaCare brings to our system? The answer is complicated, like so much about health care. Let's see what conclusions we can and cannot draw in comparison of the two systems.

As I said earlier, the VA system of healthcare is true socialized medicine. The hospitals are owned by the government. The hospital staff, and all the physicians, are employees of the federal government. The government pays all the bills – which are financed through taxes. This is very similar to the British National Health Service (NHS).

In Chapter Six, I pointed out the deficiencies of the NHS, especially with regard to waiting times for treatment. Now we see the same problem is rampant in the only true socialized medicine model in this country. The problem exists in every country where true socialized medicine is found.

The reasons are obvious. When people are given positions of responsibility without any accountability, nor incentives to perform at their best, they will do the least amount of work possible. When systems have more demand than medical resources to meet that demand, the result will always be rationing – increased waiting times to receive treatment. Tragically, the result will often be people dying while they wait.

Although ObamaCare is not a true socialized medicine system, it does create perverse incentives that will result in similar outcomes. It provides government subsidies to purchase private health insurance, however it determines what choices are available in those insurance plans. It expands Medicaid, which is a single-payer system, but does nothing to alleviate the shortage of medical providers nor the disincentives for those providers to accept Medicaid patients.

Some liberals would prefer true socialized medicine much like the VA system. Liberal *New York Times* columnist Nicholas Kristof argued for such a system during the debate before passage of the ACA in September 2009. He wrote:

"The truth is that government, for all its flaws, manages to do some things right, so that today few people doubt the wisdom of public police or firefighters. And the government has a particularly good record in medical care. Take the hospital system run by the Department of Veterans Affairs, the largest integrated health system in the United States. It is fully government run, much more 'socialized

medicine' than is Canadian health care with its private doctors and hospitals. ***And the system for veterans is by all accounts one of the best-performing and most cost-effective elements in the American medical establishment."***

I am wondering when Mr. Kristof will write his follow-up column to distance himself from those remarks now that the VA system has been so heavily criticized. Jeffrey Dorfman, writing an op-ed for *Forbes*, has a much better grasp of reality. He opines:

"The true scandal is not that people within the VA created fake waiting lists to hide the real, months-long wait which caused some veterans to die. The true scandal is that such a system was created in the first place. This is how government-provided, nationalized health care works. It budgets money for a certain amount of service and then rations that amount amongst its patients through a waiting system."

This is precisely what happens today with Medicaid, and will happen soon with Medicare, as limits on payments to providers cause rationing of health care by limited *access.* Just as the veterans must wait increasingly longer times to receive health care, so too does this occur today with Medicaid patients.

That's why studies show that people with Medicaid are 40% more likely to seek their health care in hospital emergency rooms than people without insurance. Since the non-partisan Congressional Budget Office (CBO) has estimated Medicare reimbursement rates to physicians will fall below Medicaid rates by 2020, look for the same problems of *access* to physicians to plague Medicare in the near future.

No one expects to see an ObamaCare scandal exactly like what is happening at the VA because there are no financial incentives built into the law that reward phony waiting times. But expect the same increasing delays in providing healthcare as the system increases the number of insured without increasing the number of providers.

Our veterans deserve the best healthcare possible; at least as good as other Americans enjoy. The VA system has failed them miserably but ObamaCare won't be much better. Let's fix the system for everyone soon. There's no time to waste while people die waiting for health care.

8

The Abortion Reality

"And one more misunderstanding I want to clear up - under our plan, no federal dollars will be used to fund abortions, and federal conscience laws will remain in place."
President Barack Obama
Speech to Joint Session of Congress, 9/10/09

The dirty little secret is out. ObamaCare funds abortions. That's right; despite the White House denials, even their own Government Accountability Office (GAO) confirms it is true.

You may remember in the debate in 2009 and 2010 before passage of The Affordable Care Act (ObamaCare), there were many concerns, even from Democrats, that ObamaCare would be used to fund abortions. Since the Congress needed every Democratic vote to pass the legislation (Republicans were united in their opposition), the concerns of even a few Democrats were crucial to the outcome.

Democratic Opposition

In the House of Representatives, Bart Stupak (D – MI) led a group of so-called "blue dog" Democrats who opposed funding of abortions by ObamaCare. Their opposition to this issue represented a major stumbling block for the Obama Administration in their attempts to pass the new healthcare legislation. In addition to Rep. Stupak, the group included Steve Driehaus (D – OH), Marcy Kaptur (D – OH), Nick Rahal (D – WV) Alan Mollohan (D – WV), Kathy Dahlkemper

(D – PA), Joe Donnelly (D – IN), Bobby Rush (D – IL) and Loretta Sanchez (D – CA).

The group held out for a compromise from the Obama Administration that would not violate their objections to the funding of abortions by ObamaCare.

The compromise they were looking for came just two days before the final vote on the law. On March 21, 2010, Rep. Stupak called a press conference and announced that a deal had been brokered with the White House. The deal consisted of an "executive order" from President Obama that would satisfy their concerns. He said that he would now vote for the bill and that Representatives Driehaus, Kaptur, Rahal, Mollohan, Dahlkemper, and Donnelly all agreed to the deal. Representatives Rush and Sanchez were still undecided.

In an interview on Fox News after the press conference, Stupak said the executive order was a "very strong statement" that wouldn't replace statutory language – his preference – but acknowledged that he couldn't get such language through the Senate.

"All the safeguards we were looking for, the principle we fought for all these months, will be enforced through this executive order," Stupak said. *"It's a good agreement."*

Senator Ben Nelson of Nebraska was also a vocal critic of funding abortion so the White House bribed him with the "Cornhusker Kickback"- a promise of increased Medicaid funding for the state of Nebraska and the right of states to refuse abortion coverage in the state exchanges. In return, Nelson delivered the deciding vote in the Senate that gave the Democrats a filibuster-proof majority.

Nelson explained the compromise wording of the law that he engineered in a speech on the Senate floor in 2009:

"The insurance company must bill you separately, and you must pay separately from your own personal funds – perhaps a credit card transaction, your separate personal check, or automatic withdrawal from your bank account – for that abortion coverage. Now, let me say

that again. You have to write two checks; one for the basic policy and one for the additional coverage for abortion."

This specific wording of the law was in order to comply with the Hyde Amendment, a law passed in 1976 forbidding federal funds to be used for providing abortions in the Medicaid program, except in cases of incest or rape, or when the mother's life is endangered. By separating out the payments this would ensure that only the policyholder, and not the taxpayers, would be paying for abortion coverage. Furthermore, Nelson made sure that states that did not wish to cover abortion services on their state exchanges could opt out of the program.

The President's Promise

President Obama made a promise to Congress that no federal dollars would be used to fund abortions. In a speech to the Congress on September 10, 2009, he laid out his health care reform plan. By my count there are at least 14 misrepresentations of the law that eventually became known as ObamaCare. Of these, two were made when he said this:

"And one more misunderstanding I want to clear up – under our plan, no federal dollars will be used to fund abortions, and federal conscience laws will remain in place."

The latter part of that promise was broken when Hobby Lobby had to take their case to the Supreme Court to uphold their rights of conscience. Now the GAO has revealed that the former part of that promise has also been broken.

Republican Concerns

Despite the promises of President Obama, and the reassurances of those in Congress such as Representative Stupak and Senator Nelson, Republicans wanted to be certain the spirit, as well as the law, of the Hyde Amendment would be preserved. In an attempt to permanently codify the Hyde Amendment, Rep. Chris Smith (R – N. J.) introduced legislation called the No Taxpayer Funding for Abortion and Abortion Insurance Full Disclosure Act (HR – 7) on May 14, 2013.

The bill passed the House of Representatives on January 28, 2014, by a 227-188 vote with six Democrats joining 221 Republicans.

"We are simply ensuring that hardworking Americans who pay taxes and oppose abortion don't see their taxpayer dollars going to fund abortion," said Rep. Lynn Jenkins (R – Kan.), vice chairwoman of the Republican Conference. *"We've had legislation similar to this bill in place for over three decades."* (the Hyde Amendment)

Democrats accused Republicans of waging a "war on women," designed to chip away at reproductive rights and strip women of their access to coverage through private health insurance. Some continued to deny the existence of taxpayer funding of abortion.

"There is no taxpayer funding of abortion," Rep. Diana DeGette, (D – Colo.) said. *"The Affordable Care Act does not change that."*

"This is propaganda, it's political," said Rep. Henry Waxman (D – Calif.), ranking member of the House Energy and Commerce Committee. *"The Republicans are trying to make people believe their taxpayer dollars are being used to pay for abortions. It's not true."*

This bill represents the 50th time the House has passed legislation to amend or repeal parts or all of the Affordable Care Act. Like the other bills before it, Senate Majority Leader Harry Reid has thus far refused to bring it up for a vote in the Senate.

GAO Report

The Government Accountability Office (GAO) is a non-partisan congressional research group. Recently they examined abortion coverage in the health-insurance exchanges set up for selling ObamaCare policies. Twenty-six states and the District of Columbia permit the selling of policies within these exchanges that cover abortion. In the other twenty-four states legislation was passed prohibiting the selling of any insurance plans on the exchanges that cover abortion services.

In all, they found 1036 plans that include abortion coverage, including every plan in five states: New Jersey, Connecticut, Vermont,

Rhode Island, and Hawaii. Also, more than 95% of the plans in Massachusetts, New York, and California cover abortion.

The GAO report goes on to say; *"Fifteen issuers and the Washington Health Benefit Exchange . . . did not itemize the premium amount associated with non-excepted abortion services coverage on enrollees' bills nor indicate that they send a separate bill for that premium amount."*

Timothy P. Carney, writing for *The Washington Examiner,* analyzes the report:

"The new GAO report shows that, instead, taxpayers are subsidizing abortions. Customers in five states have no abortion-free plans available to them, and in many states, customers can't tell which plans cover abortion and which don't.

In Washington State, for instance, the state's exchange bills customers on behalf of insurers- and the exchange covers abortion with federal tax dollars. The GAO found: "The exchange's billing system was not assessing any premium to individuals whose premiums are fully subsidized under the law if these individuals are enrolled in QHPs (Qualified Health Plans) that cover non-excepted abortion services."

This means customers with abortion coverage were getting their entire premium covered by federal tax credits. This is clearly an abortion subsidy – paid for by the taxpayers. This is a violation of the Hyde Amendment and a violation of the Affordable Care Act – and **another broken Obama promise.**

Carl Anderson, writing for *National Review Online,* further explains the situation:

"This report is likely to contain surprising news for the residents of these states. The GAO report makes clear that those who want to find a plan that does not cover abortion will have a very difficult time. In some cases, the information is available in the Summary of Benefits. In other cases, it is only available on the insurer's website. In other cases, the information is available only by calling the insurer."

Others say the information is unavailable – unless you first purchase the policy. Arina O. Grossu, writes that the Family Research Council has had great difficulty obtaining such information when surveying insurance companies. The explanation for this difficulty can be found in the law itself. She explains:

*"Section 1303 (b)(3)(A) of the Affordable Care Act contains a clause stating that the insurer "shall provide a notice to enrollees, **only** as part of the summary of benefits and coverage explanation, **at the time of enrollment**, of such coverage."* (emphasis added) *The law is deliberately written, in other words, to make it difficult to get this information."*

In Connecticut, after the Bracy family lost their non-ObamaCare-compliant pro-life plan, they filed a lawsuit (*Bracy v. Burwell*) in May 2014 alleging there weren't any pro-life plans available for them to purchase on the exchange. Alliance Defending Freedom (ADF), the same law firm that represented Conestoga Wood Specialties in the *Hobby Lobby v. Burwell* lawsuit that opposed the Contraception Mandate, represents them.

Three Ways Taxpayers Fund Abortion

Casey Mattox, senior counsel with ADF, notes three ways that ObamaCare is forcing taxpayers – and in some cases unwitting policyholders (maybe you) – to pay for others' abortions, steering untold millions of dollars toward Planned Parenthood and other abortion dealers. It's no coincidence that these are the same people who have been spending millions to elect President Obama and his political allies.

First, the GAO report concludes that more than 1,000 ObamaCare health insurance plans nationwide are eligible for taxpayer subsidies despite including elective abortion coverage. As previously seen in Washington, the entire premium – including the portion covering elective abortions –is being paid for by federal taxpayer dollars.

Second, the GAO confirmed that getting information on which policies cover abortion and which don't is nearly impossible. This means your plan is probably collecting an additional fee – undisclosed to you on your bill – used expressly to pay for others' abortions.

Third, the GAO report confirms that in five states, Connecticut, Rhode Island, New Jersey, Vermont, and Hawaii – it is impossible to obtain insurance plans that do not cover abortion. Thus every plan is collecting a separate fee from every enrollee to pay for others' elective abortions. Failure to purchase a plan leaves you vulnerable to the Individual Mandate tax, as well as the cost of needed healthcare services.

Mattox says that the impetus for this situation comes from Planned Parenthood, the largest provider of abortion services in this country. Planned Parenthood has increased its share of the total abortion market every year for the last three decades. It performs more than 330,000 abortions per year at an average of $468 per abortion.

This brings in approximately $150 million in abortion revenue annually, which is 38% of their health center revenue. Add to this the $500 million in annual taxpayer funding and you have a billion dollar abortion giant keenly interested in continuing this stream of revenue. No wonder they have spent tens of millions of dollars to re-elect President Obama and his supporters.

Planned Parenthood also participated widely in the enrollment process for ObamaCare. In the run-up for the open enrollment in 2013, "navigators" and "assisters" were hired by the Obama administration. Many of these people worked for Planned Parenthood. The Heritage Foundation's Sarah Torre reports the numbers:

"The Obama Administration awarded over $655,000 in taxpayer grants to Planned Parenthood affiliates in Iowa, Montana, and New Hampshire to act as "navigators", helping to enroll Americans in federally facilitated insurance exchanges. The District of Columbia awarded $375,000 – one of the largest "assister" grants in the District - to Planned Parenthood Metropolitan D.C. to help enroll citizens in the District's state-based healthcare exchange. Likewise, California, Minnesota, and Vermont have awarded a total of over $700,000 to

local Planned Parenthood affiliates to aid individuals' enrollment in their state exchanges, and many more states will likely follow suit."

Planned Parenthood is also listed as an "essential community provider" (ECP), a designation that allows them to benefit greatly from ObamaCare. The law requires that qualified insurance plans cover a sufficient number of these ECPs, defined as health care providers and hospitals that predominantly serve "low-income, medically underserved individuals." These organizations include federally qualified health clinics, hospitals, and Title X family planning centers, among other providers.

ObamaCare stipulates that in order for insurers to sell a qualified health plan on an exchange, it must cover a minimum of 10 percent to 20 percent of the ECPs in a plan's coverage area. According to a non-exhaustive list of essential community providers released by the Department of Health and Human Services, those family planning providers could include more than 400 local Planned Parenthood affiliates.

Some states, such as Minnesota, have established their own exchanges with the ability to set higher standards, including requiring insurers in their state to cover all available ECPs and the covered services they provide. In Minnesota, all health plans are required to offer contracts to all state-recognized ECPs in the insurer's coverage area. Once under contract with an ECP, insurers are required to pay for all covered benefits offered by the provider, including elective abortion services.

There can be no doubt that such provisions of the law, crafted with the input of Planned Parenthood, will serve them well financially in the years to come. Planned Parenthood Minnesota/North Dakota/ South Dakota, the largest affiliate in the state, admits it has benefitted from the state's mandate. Minnesota will maintain that requirement for health plans sold on its exchange, forcing participating insurers to offer contracts to Planned Parenthood affiliates and other abortion providers.

How Consumers Should Respond

If you are a consumer living in one of the 24 states that have passed specific legislation to prevent the selling of abortion services with insurance policies on the exchanges, you cannot purchase a policy that includes abortion coverage. If you are one of the many Americans who object to this procedure, you need not worry that your policy will be charging for this service. Nor are others in your state receiving taxpayer subsidies for abortions.

Twenty-four states restrict abortion coverage in private plans offered through health insurance marketplaces.

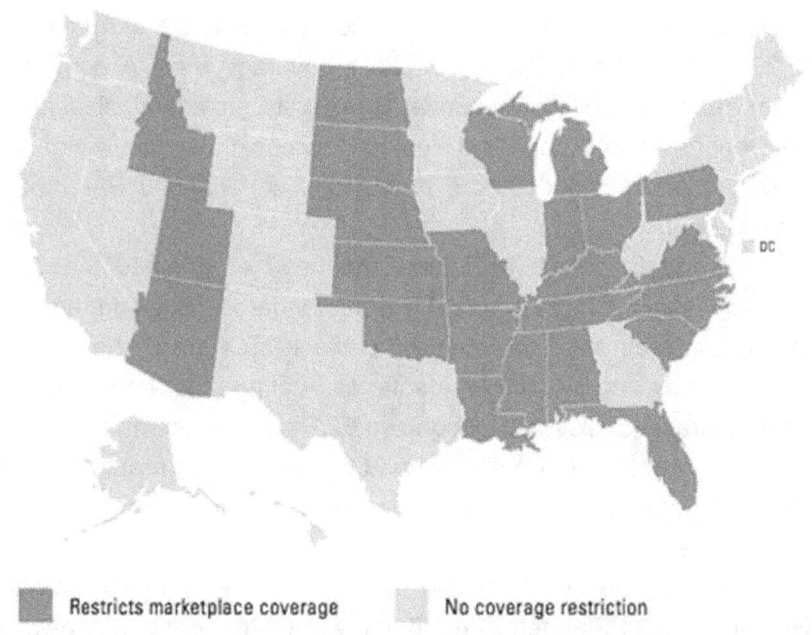

Restricts marketplace coverage   No coverage restriction

Figure 1 – Shows those states in red that restrict abortion coverage on the Exchange.

However, if you live in one of the 26 states or the District of Columbia that still allow abortion services with insurance policies sold on the exchanges, you may be paying extra for these services without your knowledge. ObamaCare requires a minimum payment of $1/month or $12/year for abortion coverage and this may not be itemized on your bill. In fact, it may be nearly impossible for you to find out if your policy provides this coverage in advance of your purchase.

If you live in one of these states or D. C., the law provides that at least one of the plans in each exchange must exclude elective abortion coverage. (Section 1334 (a)(6). But the GAO report now confirms this is not happening in at least the five states of Connecticut, New Jersey, Rhode Island, Vermont, and Hawaii.

Yet, if your policy does provide abortion services, then you certainly are being charged extra for them whether or not you intend to use them. According to a report by The Heritage Foundation,

"Everyone, regardless of sex or age, who enrolls in a federally subsidized plan that includes coverage of elective abortion will be forced to pay the separate abortion surcharge."

This leaves Americans living in one of these 26 states or D.C. with few, if any, acceptable options:

- *Enroll in a health plan that includes abortion coverage.* This means paying extra for a service you don't need and may find morally objectionable. Unfortunately, you may not even be able to discern if your policy has such coverage at all.
- *Enroll in an exchange plan or private plan that does not include abortion coverage – if one is available.* Good luck if you find yourself living in one of the five states mentioned in the GAO report above.
- *Enroll in the federally run multi-state plan that will not include abortion coverage.* One of the multi-state plans sponsored by the Office of Personnel Management (OPM) is required to exclude abortion coverage. However, such plans are only required in 60 percent of state exchanges in 2014 and won't be available in all states until 2017. This kind of coverage is only available to federal employees.

Who Will Be Supporting Abortions?

This leaves us with the important question of "Who will be supporting abortions?"

Certainly anyone paying for an insurance policy that covers abortions, whether you intend to use those services or not, will be supporting abortion through the payment of your premiums. Unfortunately, you can't be sure you're not supporting abortions just by not having a policy that provides abortion coverage.

The Heritage Foundation explains:

"Even if individuals and families successfully navigate the labyrinth of abortion-funding provisions in the exchanges and avoid covering elective abortion in their own plans, taxpayer funds will unavoidably go to fund some health plans that include such coverage. Whether through tax credits to private health plans in a state that allows abortion coverage in its exchange or through subsidies to the multi-state plans that include such coverage, taxpayers will be supporting access to plans that cover elective abortion."

The Charlotte Lozier Institute, a pro-life research organization, has analyzed this new funding for health plans that include elective abortion coverage and estimated its impact on the number of abortions performed. They conclude:

"If only one-third of the girls and women who are newly privately covered for elective abortions proceed and file for them, an additional 18,397 abortions will be paid for each year under ObamaCare's exchange expansion.

Supposedly those monies collected from the additional abortion coverage surcharge will pay for these abortions. But it is the taxpayer-funded subsidies available for all exchange health plans that will allow such coverage in the first place.

Abortifacients

There is another issue left out of this discussion that is also important. ObamaCare requires every insurance policy sold to include "essential health benefits" determined by the HHS Secretary. Former

HHS Secretary Kathleen Sebelius insisted that these benefits include contraceptives, sterilization procedures, and drugs and devices that induce abortion – known as abortifacients.

This was the central issue of the *Hobby Lobby v. Burwell* lawsuit recently decided by the Supreme Court in favor of Hobby Lobby and the other plaintiffs, Conestoga Wood Specialties and Mardel Bookstores. The High Court ruled that these plaintiffs could not be forced to provide abortifacients, which they found objectionable, to their employees because they violated their religious freedoms. The employees are still receiving contraceptives free and may purchase abortifacients with their own money, if they choose.

However, anyone else who has purchased health insurance without such coverage of these benefits is non-compliant under the provisions of the Individual Mandate and subject to a tax assessed by the IRS at the time of income tax filing. Therefore, to be compliant with the law's requirements, you must purchase a plan that provides these contraceptives and abortifacients, even if you do not intend to use them.

If you don't use them, there is no violation of your conscience. However, it should be understood, just as in the case of those who purchase policies with abortion services but do not intend to use them, you will be subsidizing those who do use them. The cost of these services is built into the premium price of your policy and no deduction will be given even if you don't intend to use them. There are no plans available without them, unless you've been granted a waiver such as the employees at Hobby Lobby.

Once again, the Heritage Foundation makes this clear:

"All health insurance offered on state exchanges must meet new federal standards for "qualified health plans". The law's preventive services mandate requires that all qualified health plans cover – without co-pay, deductible, or other charge to the enrollee – abortion-inducing drugs and devices, contraception, sterilization, and related education and counseling. All individuals and families obtaining health care coverage on any state's exchange will participate in and pay for plans that include coverage of those drugs and services."

How to Protect Life and Conscience

What is the solution to this dilemma for those who object to abortions and abortifacients? Must they accept the fact that their tax dollars will go to subsidize these morally objectionable procedures even though they abstain from their use themselves?

Once again, I am indebted to the Heritage Foundation for clarification of the solutions to this moral quagmire. They suggest the following options:

- **States should prohibit abortion coverage on their exchanges.** The 26 states and the District of Columbia without "opt-out" laws should pass legislation prohibiting insurers from offering coverage of elective abortion on their exchanges. Such reform would prevent taxpayer subsidies from flowing to these plans and protect individuals and families form being forced to pay a separate abortion premium if they should find themselves enrolled in a plan that covers abortion.

- **Congress should permanently prohibit federal abortion funding.** At the federal level, congress can enact broad protections against taxpayer funding of abortion and abortion coverage. The No Taxpayer Funding for Abortion Act (H.R. 7), for example, would ensure that "*no funds authorized or appropriated by federal law*" could be used to pay for abortion or health benefit plans that cover abortion. This would simply continue the principle of the Hyde Amendment, which has been in routine use in this country for nearly forty years.

- **Congress should protect the right of conscience.** Congress can also enact protections for individuals, employers, and issuers from being forced to offer, provide, or pay for coverage of drugs and services that violate their deeply held moral or religious beliefs. Likewise, Congress should codify across federal law protections for the rights of conscience of health care insurers, providers, and personnel who decline to provide, pay for, provide coverage of, or refer for abortions.

- **Defund and repeal ObamaCare.** To truly protect taxpayers, individuals, and families, ObamaCare must be repealed in its entirety. Until then, Congress should focus on defunding, delaying, and dismantling the health care law to make room for real reform.

There are better ways of providing health care that do not create these moral dilemmas and still ensure high quality, lower cost, health care for all Americans. We will discuss these in detail in Chapter Twelve.

9

The Cost of ObamaCare –
Economic Reality

"Today we've seen a dramatic slowdown in the rising cost of health care."
President Barack Obama
Speech at Northwestern University, 10/2/14

President Barack Obama took another victory lap. In a speech at Northwestern University to commemorate the one-year anniversary of the opening of enrollment for the Affordable Care Act, he elected to spin the law's achievements. Considering the disastrous experience of the law's rollout the year before, you might have expected some humility.

But not this president. Obama took advantage of the occasion to claim the law was responsible for "*a dramatic slowdown in the rising cost of health care.*"

How true is this claim? Is it correct to say there has been a dramatic slowdown in the rising cost of health care and, if so, should ObamaCare be given the credit?

The president went on to claim credit for "*an $1800 tax credit*" for every American family as a result of ObamaCare. Is this statement true and accurate?

In this chapter we will explore these and other questions regarding the economic impact of ObamaCare. We will look at the impact it has had on the costs of healthcare and what other factors may be contributing to that impact. Only when we have answered these questions will we be able to judge the true cost of this legislation on our economy and the future fiscal stability of our country.

The Impact on Health Care Costs

Everyone knows that health care costs have been rising rapidly for decades. Every business owner recognizes this truth when he or she writes the checks to pay for employee health care. Every patient knows this when they pay the deductibles at their doctor's office.

Health care costs have been rising faster than inflation for a long time. After a slowdown in the early 1990s, some concluded we finally had healthcare costs under control. But the late 1990s brought back healthcare inflation and annual healthcare spending grew to 9.7 percent by 2002, renewing fears of future bankruptcy if the pattern continued.

But this pattern changed early after the start of the new millennium.

In 2002, health care expenditures peaked at a rate of 9.7% according to the Centers for Medicare and Medicaid Services (CMS). The following year, 2003, began a decline in the rate of growth, which has continued thereafter for ten straight years, leveling off at 3.7% in 2012 and then rising again gradually. This downward trend began *seven years before passage of ObamaCare* and eleven years before implementation of the law beginning in 2014.

Yet, the Obama administration wants to attribute these declines to the Affordable Care Act. This was a major selling point of the new healthcare law in 2010. Peter Orszag, President Obama's budget director, insisted the new healthcare law entitlement would actually improve America's long-run fiscal position by revolutionizing the delivery of medical care.

To be sure, the outlook for the future has improved, at least for now. The Centers for Medicare and Medicaid Services (CMS) projected in 2010 that U.S. healthcare spending in 2019 would be $4.5 Trillion. This year they revised this number down to $4.0 Trillion, a savings of $500 Billion. The White House believes ObamaCare gets the credit.

However, the first quarter of 2014 saw an astounding increase of spending to 9.9 percent. That's the largest percent change in the rate of healthcare spending since 1980. Opponents of ObamaCare want to blame ObamaCare for this increase. John C. Goodman, healthcare economist, says neither conclusion is correct.

Goodman documents the downward trend of health care spending that started long before ObamaCare started (Figure 1), but also acknowledges it is too soon for ObamaCare to be blamed for the upward movement in spending in the first quarter of 2014. Goodman explains:

"It's too soon for ObamaCare to have resulted in a big boost in spending. And the previous slowdown was underway over a decade. Over the longer period, what does track the slowdown very closely are three other developments: the growth of Health Savings Accounts (HSAs), the growth of Health Reimbursement Accounts (HRAs) and the general trend toward higher deductibles. All three changes mean that patients are paying more medical bills out of their own pockets. And that has produced profound changes – both on the demand and the supply side of the market."

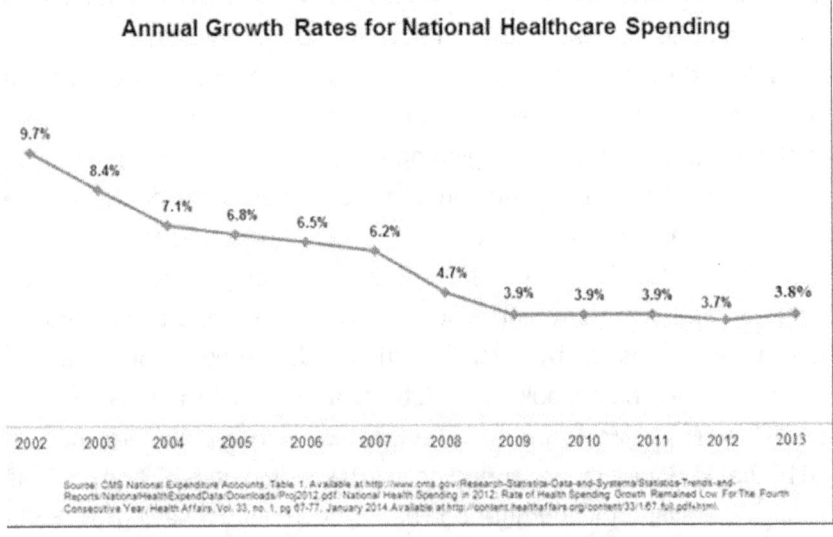

Figure 1 – Annual Growth Rates for National Healthcare Spending – 2002 – 2013. Source: Center for Medicare and Medicaid Services – CMS.gov

HSAs, HRAs, and other high deductible healthcare insurance policies all contribute to lowering healthcare costs by increasing the incentive for patients to delay health care treatment. When patients bear some of the costs of medical decisions, they participate more in the decision-making process. Studies have shown the use of these plans can lower costs by as much as 30%.

Why did healthcare costs begin going down in 2003?

Two important changes took place in 2003. The opportunity to have an HSA plan was created by legislation in Congress in 2003. Participation in HSAs has grown steadily since that time. In 2012 they grew by 22% with total HSA assets soaring to nearly $15.5 billion. Goodman says there has been a parallel growth in HRA plans, a similar arrangement commonly offered by large employers. Today, nearly 30 million Americans are covered by these consumer-driven health plans.

Enrollment in consumer-driven health plans now exceeds enrollment in HMOs. According to the Kaiser Family Foundation survey, one-fifth of all workers are now enrolled in these plans, up from 8% in 2008. As these individual accounts have grown, national health spending growth has slowed.

The other change that took place was the passage of the Medicare Modernization Act of 2003. This change in Medicare by President George W. Bush created Medicare Advantage plans and Medicare Part D, a new prescription-drug benefit for seniors.

Reihan Salam, writing in *National Review,* says this lowered health care costs because of the popularity of the Medicare Advantage Plans (MA). Unlike regular Medicare, called Medicare FFS, in which the federal government reimburses healthcare providers for each service rendered, Medicare Advantage is administered by private insurance companies and health-care organizations. They receive a fixed payment from the federal government for each patient.

ObamaCare actually calls for a reduction in these plans and has cut reimbursement rates to the insurance companies. Many expected this to reduce the popularity of these plans but enrollment is actually growing. Facing reduced payments, MA plans have had to cut costs, including narrowing the provider networks (reducing the number of physicians available on the network). These adjustments have allowed them to offer lower monthly premiums. As of 2013, 28 percent of Medicare beneficiaries were enrolled in these plans. There seems to be a growing number of seniors, especially those on fixed incomes, who choose these plans.

ObamaCare was supposed to cut the funding of these plans by another $156 billion but President Obama delayed these cuts until after the mid-term elections. Yet, ironically, studies show these plans actually save the taxpayers money. A 2012 study published in *The Journal of the American Medical Association* compared Medicare FFS and Medicare Advantage plans and found that the MA plans can deliver the same package of benefits for 10 percent less cost than Medicare FFS on average.

The MA plans are achieving these cost savings by adopting integrated managed-care systems through a trial-and-error process. In contrast, the Obama administration has been promoting provider integration through ObamaCare's tightly regulated Accountable Care Organizations (ACOs). These ACOs offer providers incentives to organize care in specific ways prescribed by the federal government. Yet these ACOs are failing to see the same savings found in the MA plans. (More on ACOs later)

The second part of the Medicare Modernization Act of 2003 created Medicare Part D, a new prescription drug benefit for seniors. Because this plan incentivizes the use of generic drugs that lower costs, the plan has contributed to lower overall healthcare spending more than had been anticipated. Prescription-drug use reduces other health costs, especially hospitalization and therefore deserves much of the credit for the downward trend in healthcare spending.

Another reason for the decline in spending over the last decade is the willingness of employers to switch to high-deductible insurance plans. As employers try to cut their rising healthcare costs, they choose plans for their employees that pass more of the cost onto them. These high-deductible plans have built-in disincentives for their employees to seek medical attention except when really necessary. By passing along more of the up-front costs of healthcare, employers reduce overall healthcare spending.

Another factor contributing to the continued decline in annual healthcare spending is the recession. While the slowdown in healthcare spending began in 2003, when the economy was robust, the recession brought on by the collapse of the financial markets in 2008 brought further declines. The annual growth rate of spending was essentially flat from 2005 to 2007, declining only from 6.8 percent to 6.2 percent in three years. But with the 2008 recession, annual health care spending growth took a steeper decline to 4.7 percent. It has continued to decline since 2008 although leveling off at about 3.9 percent annually through 2013.

Even the left-leaning Kaiser Family Foundation analysis in 2013 concluded the slowdown in the growth of spending could be attributed to the economy. Here's what they said:

"Based on statistical analysis of 50 years of health spending and economic trends, the study finds that the economy, including factors such as Gross Domestic Product growth and inflation, produces a major but delayed effect on the nation's health spending. This effect stretches over a period of six years, meaning that the recession that ended in 2009 will continue to dampen health care spending for several more years and that spending will increase gradually as the economy strengthens."

With the first quarter 2014 rate of growth rising to 9.9 percent on an annualized basis, it seems that the decline in healthcare spending is over. It is too soon to know if this is an aberrant blip on the radar or an alarming trend. But the real costs of ObamaCare can't be measured accurately until the costs for the insurance bailout are calculated and the real cost of health insurance premiums are known. As explained in Chapter Five, we won't know these numbers until 2017 when the "3Rs", reinsurance, risk adjustments, and risk corridors expire.

What about President Obama's claim of an "$1800 tax credit"?

It's interesting that the president would try to tell us that we've all received an "$1800 tax credit." Here's the exact wording of his claim:

"If your family gets your health care through your employer, premiums are rising at a rate tied for the lowest on record. What this means for the economy is staggering. If we hadn't taken this on, and premiums had kept growing at the rate they did in the last decade, the average premium for family coverage today would be $1800 higher than they are. That's $1800 you don't have to pay out of our pocket or see vanish from your paycheck. That's like a $1800 tax cut."

First of all, notice how his previous claim about ObamaCare's impact has changed:

"We'll lower premiums by up to $2500 for a typical family per year. . . We'll do it by the end of my first term as president of the United States." (June 5, 2008)

That promise failed to materialize. According to Kaiser Family Foundation/HRET Employer Health Benefits Survey, average premiums for family coverage were $13,375 in 2009 and $16,531 in 2013. This means average premiums for family coverage *rose* by $2,976 by the end of President Obama's first term. Therefore the direction and the magnitude of the impact on family insurance premiums was the opposite of what the president promised.

Now he wants to brag that he's actually lowered our premiums by $1800 per family, though he doesn't mention his former promise that it would be $2500. Unfortunately, the facts just don't support either statement. In my last book, *The ObamaCare Train Wreck,* I addressed this very issue. I've reproduced that portion of the book here:

In an effort to spin this failure the White House has tried to argue that the president meant that premiums would be $2500 less than they would have been otherwise if not for ObamaCare. This suggestion that the new law would "bend the cost curve down" is also false. For three consecutive years, the Office of the Actuary at CMS (Medicare/Medicaid) has released 10 year projections that compare national health spending under ObamaCare with spending assuming ObamaCare had never been implemented. Each year the ACA increases aggregate national health spending above and beyond the amount that such spending would have increased otherwise.

Chris Conover explains: *"The latest version of these projections, released just last month (September 2013), shows that between 2010 and 2022, aggregate health spending will be $621 Billion higher under the ObamaCare scenario. For a typical family of four, this amounts to $7,579 over that 13 year period."*

Rather than lower expectations on this promise, Obama doubled-down on this extravagant claim. On July 16, 2012, he assured small business owners that *"your premiums will go down."* This assertion, despite the fact that the Medicare actuaries had demonstrated that the ACA would *increase* healthcare spending. The Washington Post fact-checker awarded this claim with Three Pinocchios. (Significant factual error and/or obvious contradictions)

Patrick Brennan, writing for *National Review,* also found this latest Obama claim unsubstantiated:

"First, this is only like an $1800 tax cut if you expect your taxes to rise, say, 8 to 10 percent a year, as health insurance premiums often do – Americans are not seeing premiums drop for comparable employer health plans. Premiums have risen relatively slowly for employer plans over the past couple years, but there's almost no way the president can possibly claim credit for this. The Affordable Care Act didn't "take on" employer health insurance at all, really – it only made small, relatively inexpensive tweaks to that market (such as the HHS mandate).

Employer premiums are rising slowly for a couple reasons: the overall health-cost slowdown and the continued shift to high-deductible, health-savings-account plans. The latter is due in large part to President Bush's Medicare Modernization Act of 2003, which made such savings accounts much more feasible. (ObamaCare's Cadillac tax will also drive the growth of these plans in the future – he does deserve credit for that.)"

Update on Premium Increases

Conover updated his previous comments with a new analysis of premium costs based, not on projections, but on real numbers. The Society of Actuaries estimated in 2013 that the ACA would result in increasing claims costs by an average of 32 percent nationally by 2017. Numerous studies showed there had been double-digit increases in premiums when comparing actual Exchange premiums to previously-prevailing premiums in the non-group market. But such projections were dismissed by proponents of ObamaCare since actual premiums in the Exchanges had not yet been announced.

But now comes a new study from the non-partisan National Bureau of Economic Research, published by The Brookings Institution (a liberal think-tank), that overcomes the limitations of these prior studies by examining what happened to premiums in the entire non-group market.

Conover explains:

*"In 2014, **premiums in the non-group market grew by 24.4% compared to what they would have been without ObamaCare.** Of equal importance, this careful state-by-state assessment showed that premiums rose in all but 6 states (including Washington, D.C.)."*

Unlike virtually all other studies that have been conducted to date, this new study examined premium data from both exchange and non-Exchange plans, providing a picture of the complete non-group market rather than one segment. This is crucially important since in nearly one-third of states (16), Exchange coverage constitutes 40% or less of the entire non-group market.

Critics have dismissed other studies by saying premiums in the non-group market have always gone up by a large amount, thereby exempting ObamaCare from responsibility for the increases. But this study isolates the causal impact of ObamaCare by using trend data in each state to figure out what non-group premiums in 2014 *would have been* in the absence of ObamaCare.

All of the percentage changes shown in the Figure 2 below represent the net change attributable to ObamaCare after accounting for all the other factors that would have made premiums go up. The adverse impact of ObamaCare on non-group premiums varies considerably from state to state. But the law is estimated to result in lower premiums in only 6 states. Data is incomplete, however, in two states – California and New Jersey – due to anomalous data reporting requirements. Therefore, the large estimated decline of premiums in New Jersey may be inaccurate.

Obamacare Caused Premiums To Rise in All But 6 States in 2014

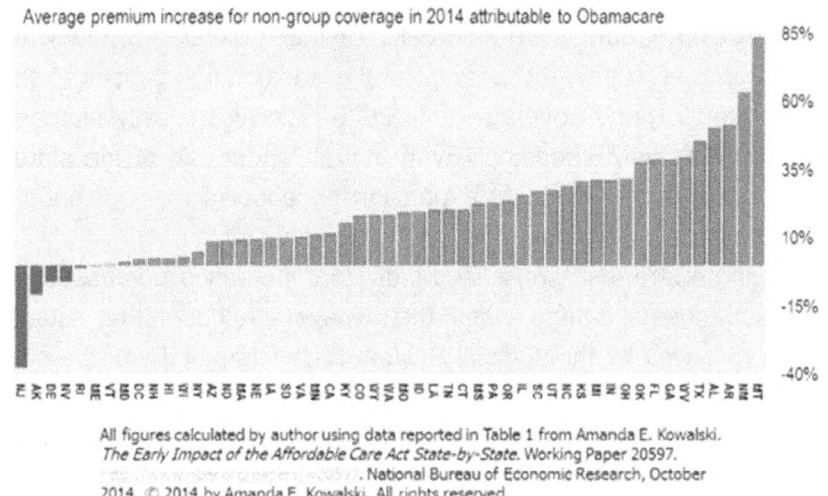

Average premium increase for non-group coverage in 2014 attributable to Obamacare

Figure 2 – The impact of ObamaCare on premiums in the states.

Note that premium increases exceed 35% in 9 states, including Oklahoma, Florida, Georgia, West Virginia, Texas, Alabama, Arkansas, New Mexico, and Montana. Conover stresses these increases are *above and beyond normal premium trends*. No one can credibly claim that these massive premium increases would have happened anyway since the study was specifically designed to isolate the law's impacts from all the other factors that have driven up premiums in recent years.

While many of these individuals may be eligible for subsidies on the Exchanges, those ineligible for subsidies will never see their premiums go down as promised by President Obama. Conover estimates that 6.2 million in the non-group market had to absorb these premium increases without the benefit of any help from the federal government.

What impact will ObamaCare have on healthcare spending?

ObamaCare was supposed to reduce healthcare spending. The law calls for a reduction in Medicare payments to providers (doctors and hospitals) of $716 Billion over the next ten years. That's an average of $71.6 Billion less spending on Medicare alone per year.

However, ObamaCare also calls for the expansion of Medicaid and promises to pay 100 percent of the additional expenses to the states that expand coverage until 2020. This will greatly increase federal healthcare spending. Even though about half of the states have refused this Medicaid expansion because of fears of budget disasters, the cost for the other half will be substantial.

ObamaCare also subsidizes individual insurance purchased on the exchanges at a huge cost to the taxpayers. Although that issue is being reviewed by the Judicial System (See Chapter Two), the cost for these subsidies is Billions of taxpayer dollars.

The cost of Medicaid expansion and tax credits for low to moderate income Americans is expected to greatly exceed any cost savings in Medicare. Furthermore, the savings in Medicare are being delayed by the Obama administration for political reasons and will not be realized anytime soon. The latest CBO estimate now calls for about $1 Trillion in additional federal deficit over the next ten years as a result of ObamaCare. This would have been much greater except for the large tax increases that come with this new healthcare legislation.

This brings us to another broken Obama promise. Here's how I described this in my earlier book:

Obama's promise: *"I can make a firm pledge under my plan, no family making less than $250,000 a year will see any form of tax increase. Not your income tax, not your payroll tax, not your capital gains taxes, not any of your taxes."* (September 12, 2008)
Reality: Conover writes: *"By 2022, Obamacare will have imposed just over $1 Trillion in new taxes. It's true that $318 Billion of this will come in the form of taxes on payroll, dividends, capital gains, and other investment income specifically targeting taxpayers earning over $200,000 (singles) or $250,000 (married)."*

Simply doing the math you can see that about $700 Billion in new taxes will come from those individuals earning less than $250,000, the ceiling that Obama said would protect middle and low-income taxpayers. *That's 70% of the new taxes.*

According to columnist Robert Allen Bonelli, ObamaCare imposes twenty hidden new taxes. *Seven of these affect all taxpayers regardless of income.* These include the **Individual Mandate tax**, now properly called a tax rather than a penalty. Then there is the **Medicine Cabinet tax**, which prohibits reimbursement of OTC medicines from your HSA, FSA, or HRA accounts (as was previously allowed). There is also the **Flexible Spending Account (FSA) Cap**, which now limits to $2500 the amount of pre-tax dollars you can shelter in these accounts.

There is also the **Medical Itemized Deduction Hurdle**, which limits the deduction of medical expenses when you file your tax return. There is a **Health Savings Account (HSA) Withdrawal Tax Hike**, an **Indoor Tanning Services Tax** and **The Cadillac Plan Tax,** an excise tax on so-called Cadillac health insurance plans of 40%, which will severely curb the use of these plans in the future. There is the **Tax on Medical Device Manufacturers** of 2.3%, which will be passed on to consumers purchasing various medical devices such as mobility assistance devices, personal testing supplies, catheters, and other medical consumer products. This tax will also have a huge impact on employment in an industry employing 360,000 people in 6,000 plants today. This tax will raise costs and lower profitability, which will result in fewer jobs.

One of the largest taxes of ObamaCare is the **Health Insurance Tax** (HIT), which is imposed on insurance companies based on their market share. Companies are expected to collectively pay $8 Billion in the HIT in 2014 according to the National Center for Policy Analysis, with collections rising to $14.3 Billion in 2018. This tax will be passed on to consumers in the form of higher premiums. Consulting firm Oliver Wyman conducted a study that found that the HIT would increase health insurance premiums by more than $2,800 per person and $6,800 per family over the next ten years.

There is also the **Reinsurance Tax** of $63 per health insurance recipient, which insurers will have to pay to the government to create a "slush fund" to bail-out those insurance companies adversely affected by ObamaCare.

There is also a 3.8% surtax, the **Capital Gains Tax,** which is assessed on capital gains and dividends for couples earning above $250,000 and individuals earning above $200,000. There is a **Medicare Wage Tax** increase of 0.9% that was imposed in 2013 which is expected to raise $317 Billion over ten years.

Conover summarizes the reality thus: *"In short, when all is said and done, the very folks the president assured wouldn't see taxes go up a dime to bankroll health reform will shoulder close to 70 percent of ObamaCare's tax burden. The president has shown himself to be a diligent student of former Louisiana Senator Russell Long: "Don't tax you, don't tax me, tax that fellow behind the tree."*

Increased government spending is always accompanied by increased taxes. It was the deceit of President Obama, and the naiveté of the American electorate that believed him, that allowed him to claim he would not raise taxes on the middle class.

The Impact of Medical Mergers

Recently there has been a trend in the medical industry for hospitals to acquire physician practices, converting these physicians into hospital employees. According to a survey of the American Hospital Association, the number of physicians working for hospitals has grown 34% in the last ten years. Nearly one out of every two doctors now works for a hospital.

Doctors make the change to rid themselves of the paperwork and stress of managing an office. With ever increasing demands on their time for documentation of everything they do, many doctors gladly choose to let a hospital handle these headaches. In exchange, they give up autonomy and focus on practicing medicine.

Hospitals particularly like the change because they can bill more for the same services of the physician if provided in a hospital setting. Fees may increase as much as 70% under the Medicare fee schedule. Hospitals enjoy a windfall as a result of these mergers.

But what happens to the cost of healthcare? No surprise – it goes up! Suzanne Delbanco, a physician and executive director of Catalyst for Payment Reform documents these changes in a *Wall Street Journal* article. She says payments to hospitals on behalf of the privately insured are an estimated 3% higher as a result of consolidation between hospitals and doctors. Lest you think this is a small number, remember we are talking about 3% of almost $900 Billion in U.S. spending on hospital care each year. That's a big number!

She gives examples: When two competing San Francisco Bay Area hospitals – Summit and Alta Bates – merged in 1999, hospital prices increased 28% – 44%, according to an analysis by the Federal Trade Commission economist Steven Tenn.

What role does ObamaCare play in these mergers?

Under the ACA, new models for delivering care, such as **Accountable Care Organizations (ACOs)**, require doctors and hospitals to work together to coordinate and improve patient care and reduce spending. Some providers contend that mergers let them achieve economies of scale and improve efficiency, enabling them to decrease costs and improve care.

But there is no evidence to support such claims. Studies show that when mergers happen in already concentrated markets, price increases can exceed 20 percent. A 2012 research study by the FTC and University of Pennsylvania professor Robert Town showed this. They also found that *"physician-hospital consolidation has not led to either improved quality or reduced costs."*

Like so much of ObamaCare, good intentions have not led to good results. Hospital mergers with physicians, encouraged by the ACA, are another contributing factor to the rising cost of healthcare.

To summarize this section, it is true that the *rate of growth* of healthcare spending has declined in recent years, but not because of ObamaCare. It began slowing in 2003 and slowed further after the recession began in 2008 for the reasons discussed above. But there is evidence to suggest this decline in the rate of growth of spending is over.

To be sure, the actual costs continue to rise, not fall. According to Dan Munro, writing for *Forbes,* the CMS projected National Health Expenditures (NHE) for 2013 are $2.9 Trillion, for 2014 $3.1 Trillion, and for 2015, $3.3 Trillion. But the Deloitte Center for Health Solutions calculates a substantially higher number when figuring in the costs of the Sustainable Growth Rate (SGR) – the so-called "doc fix" that calculates Medicare fees for doctors, as well as other direct and indirect costs.

The Deloitte Study adjusts the projections for 2013 to $3.65 Trillion, for 2014 to $3.83 Trillion, and for 2015 to $4.01 Trillion. These are substantially higher figures than the federal government numbers projected by CMS.

An Unfolding Fiscal Disaster

How will all this affect our nation's fiscal future?

President Obama said, *"I will not sign a plan that adds one dime to our deficits."* (September 9, 2009)

This pledge actually was not given in a campaign speech but rather to a joint session of Congress. He based this fiction on the scoring of the law by the CBO, which was forced to use misleading statistical information to produce the desired financial result.

The CBO was told to score the economic impact on the federal deficit using ten years of income but only six years of expenses. Congressman Paul Ryan, current chairman of the House Budget Committee, described the Obama plan as "full of gimmicks and smoke-and-mirrors" many weeks before the bill passed. His analysis showed the law would cost $2.3 Trillion over the next ten years instead of the slightly less than $1 Trillion the CBO had concluded based on the faulty data.

Others agreed with Ryan. Former CBO director Douglas Holtz-Eakin and Michael Ramet of the American Action Forum wrote, *"A more comprehensive and realistic projection suggests that the new reform law will raise the deficit by more than $500 Billion during the first ten years and by nearly $1.5 Trillion in the following decade."*

Conover points out in the follow-up article that the General Accountability Office (GAO) has shown that the ACA has put us on a path to add $6.2 *Trillion* (2011 dollars) to the deficit over the next 75 years.

Charles Blahous, director of the Spending and Budget Initiative, a senior research fellow at the Mercatus Center at George Mason University and a public trustee for Social Security and Medicare, has great concerns for our future. He describes the Affordable Care Act thus:

"It is quite possible that the ACA is shaping up as the greatest act of fiscal irresponsibility ever committed by federal legislators. Nothing immediately comes to mind as comparable to it. Certainly no tax legislation is, because tax rates rise and fall frequently, such that one Congress's tax cut can be (and often is) undone by a later tax increase. The same is true for legislation affecting appropriated spending programs. But the ACA is a commitment to permanently subsidize comprehensive health insurance for millions who could not otherwise afford it, which the federal government has no viable plan to finance. Moreover, experience show that it is very difficult to scale back such spending once large numbers of Americans have been made dependent on it."

He compares the entitlement spending of Social Security, Medicare, and Medicaid, with the ACA (Figure 3). Current fiscal problems stem from these three other entitlements whose costs continue to rise well beyond original projections. Now comes the ACA to add to our fiscal challenges.

Blahous is particularly concerned about the financing of the ACA (ObamaCare). The fiscal solvency of the law was based on certain expected sources of revenue but these are already falling apart. Among these sources are:

- **CLASS** – The ACA's "CLASS" program (Community Living Assistance and Supports) was originally projected to generate $37 Billion in net premiums through 2015 ($86 Billion over ten years). CLASS was later suspended due to its long-term financial unworkability, meaning these revenues have not materialized and will not.

Average Total Federal Deficits, Years 0 - 5 After Enactment
As a Percentage of GDP

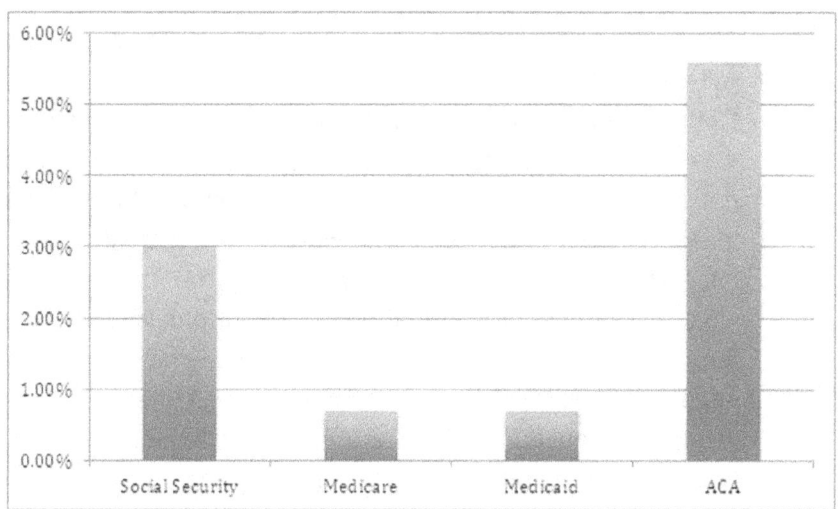

Figure 3 – How the ACA compares to other entitlement spending as a percentage of Gross Domestic Product (GDP)

- **Employer/Individual Mandate penalties** – These were supposed to have brought in $12 Billion through 2015, $101 Billion over the first ten years. Because the Obama Administration has repeatedly delayed their enforcement, to date they haven't brought in much of anything. Some ACA advocates are even beginning to downplay the significance of possibly ditching these mandates altogether, though they were central to the law's financing scheme.

- **Medicare Advantage** – The ACA was supposed to be financed in part by cuts to Medicare Advantage (MA) totaling $31 Billion through 2015, $128 Billion over the first ten years. The White House recently announced that planned MA cuts will not go into effect after all.
- **Reinsurance and Risk Corridors** – These provisions of the law were actually expected by the CBO to produce net revenues of $8 Billion for the government through the taxes imposed to pay for them. However, President Obama has already changed the provisions of the law (without Congressional approval) that control these provisions, using them as a "slush fund" to bailout insurance companies and keep insurance premiums artificially lower. Effectively, the insurance industry received an $8 billion tax break from the Obama administration. The result of these changes of the law may well produce a net negative impact on the budget.
- **Other controversial provisions** – The ACA's most controversial savings provisions – among them its ambitious Medicare provider payment reductions, the tax on so-called "Cadillac" health plans, and cost saving decisions of the Independent Payment Advisory Board – have yet to be tested. Given that less-controversial provisions have failed to meet their savings targets, there is little basis for confidence that these more controversial ones will do so.
- **Accountable Care Organizations** – One of the provisions of the ACA that was supposed to lower costs was the formation of Accountable Care Organizations (ACOs). These cooperative partnerships between hospitals and doctors were supposed to incentivize these providers to lower costs by paying them bonuses if they kept spending below established benchmarks. However, recent reports in *The Wall Street Journal* indicate these ACO experiments have been largely a bust.

  The Medicare "Pioneer" ACO project originally featured 32 experienced health systems hand-selected by HHS because they had already made progress toward the ACO model. Thirteen – or one-third of the program – have since dropped out as they spent more than the old status quo. In year one, spending increased at 14 sites and only 13 of the 32 qualified for a bonus. In year two, spending increased at six of the remaining 23 and 11 received a bonus.

After netting out the bonuses and penalties, the Pioneer ACOs saved taxpayers a grand total of $17.89 million in 2012 and $43.36 million in 2013. All in, per capita spending was a mere 0.45% lower compared to ordinary fee-for-service Medicare. Yet the upfront start-up investments for the pioneers (in administration, compliance and information technology) ran to $64 million, so at best the program is a wash.

The editorial board of *The Wall Street Journal* says,

"ACOs are failing because HHS's regulations are a classic case of counterproductive and arbitrary central planning: The government is paying hospital groups to generate slightly lower bills. As the quitters may have discovered, it is more remunerative to stay with the old system, with higher hospital bills but no bonuses."

Blahous likens the situation to imagining the impact if the Roosevelt Administration of 1937 had successfully sold the American public on the value of Social Security and promised to pay for it with a 2% payroll tax on earnings. Then, just before imposing the tax, they decided to roll back the tax while leaving in place what eventually proved to be the single most expensive spending program in the history of the American public. The result would have been a fiscal disaster of unprecedented magnitude.

That's precisely what is happening with the ACA. The public is already receiving the benefits through expansion of Medicaid and taxpayer subsidies of most individuals (87%) purchasing insurance on the exchanges. But the means of paying for these entitlements have been sharply cut back.

He says the CBO currently estimates that the ACA's coverage provisions will cost the federal government $92 Billion a year by FY2015. This is roughly 0.5 percent of projected U.S. economic output for 2015, well exceeding the relative costs of Social Security, Medicare, and Medicaid at a similar point in their history. Worse, the federal fiscal position was far weaker when the ACA was passed than when Social Security, Medicare, and Medicaid were created.

But the real trouble is in the years to come. He says the start-up costs of the ACA represent only the tip of the fiscal iceberg that will be the fully phased-in law. CBO projects that its annual costs will hit $200 Billion by FY2020, or nearly 0.9 percent of GDP. Yet this assumes that lawmakers will be content to allow the ACA's health insurance subsidies to grow more slowly than low-income beneficiaries' health care costs, as the law now stipulates. Thus there is every reason to believe that the ACA's eventual costs will far exceed initial estimates - as happened with Social Security, Medicare, and Medicaid.

10

The Impact on Jobs and Innovation

"The new health law is discouraging a significant number of firms from hiring and is also pushing workers into part-time, rather than full time jobs."
Economist John C. Goodman - 8/25/14

"The cumulative effects of the ACA could create a sect of Americans perpetually underemployed and increasingly dependent upon the government."
Congressman Bill Cassidy (R – LA) - 9/17/14

Sometimes we focus on the wrong information. In January 2009, when President Obama took the oath of office, the *unemployment rate* was 7.8 percent. It would rise to 10.0 percent by October of the same year before leveling off and beginning to decline. It would be two full years before the rate fell below 9.0 percent when it reached 8.8 percent in October of 2011. In October 2014, the rate fell to below six percent (5.9 %) for the first time since July 2008. In February, 2015 it is 5.5 percent.

Surely this is progress. Yet there is an even more important labor statistic that is only rarely discussed but a better reflection of the strength of the job market. I'm referring to the *labor force participation rate*.

Labor Force Participation Rate

When President Obama began his term of office in 2009, the labor force participation rate was 65.7 percent. When the recession ended in June 2009 the labor force participation rate was still 65.7 percent. But then it began a steady decline. In 2014 the labor force participation rate fell to 62.7 percent, the lowest rate since 1978 (Figure 1). In February, 2015 it is the same. That's a drop of three full percentage points since Obama took office. In real numbers that represents nearly 8 million workers.

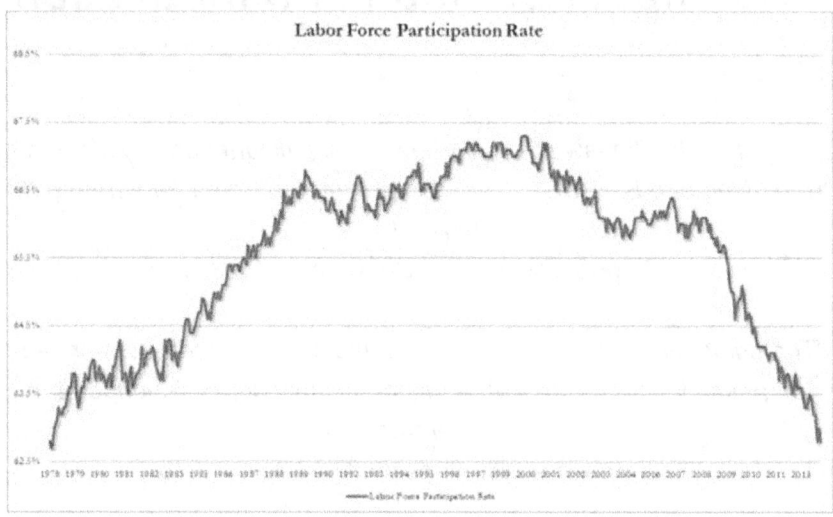

Figure 1 – Labor force participation rate from 1978 to 2014

It is important to understand that when the labor force participation rate goes down, fewer people are looking for work. They have given up trying to find a job. The job market is so bleak that they accept the fact there are no jobs out there and they settle for government assistance. That's bad for them – but good for the government! When they stop looking for work they are no longer counted in the statistics used for determining the unemployment rate. Therefore the unemployment rate goes down even though they didn't find a job.

Therefore, the White House can brag about the declining unemployment rate but there are actually fewer Americans employed. If the labor force participation rate rose to 65.7 percent, where it was when President Obama took office in 2009, the unemployment rate would actually still be above 10 percent (Figure 2).

You won't hear the White House referring to the labor force participation rate because it doesn't support their narrative that the economy is improving. But even liberal media such as *The Atlantic* grudgingly concedes the point. Jordan Weissmann writes:

"The workforce participation is an important figure because it tells us details about the job market that the ordinary old unemployment rate tends to obscure. When the Labor Department tabulates its data, it only counts adults as "unemployed" if they don't have a job but are still hunting for one. People who have given up searching for work get left out of the equation. So if enough people get discouraged by the barren labor market and stop looking for jobs, the unemployment rate, perversely enough, goes down."

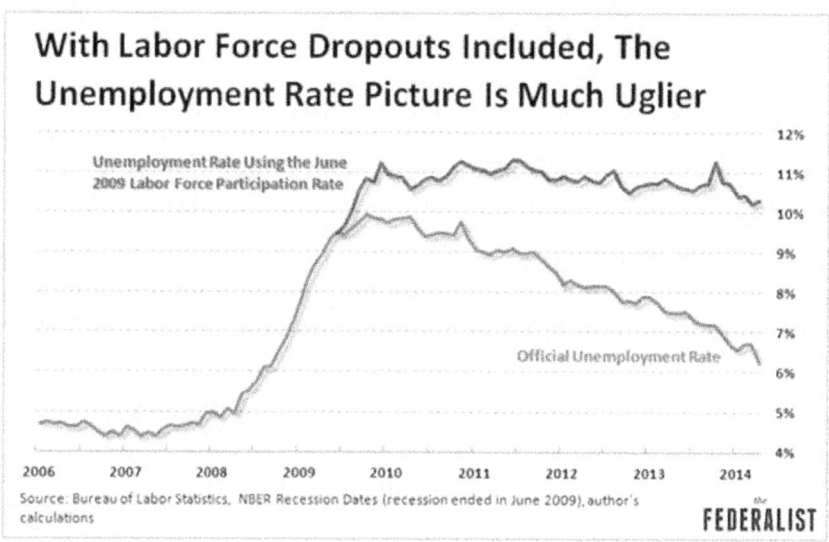

Figure 2 – Unemployment rate using 2009 Labor Force Participation Rate

Economists agree this has been the slowest recovery from a recession since the Great Depression of the 1930s. According to economist Peter Ferrara, contributor to *Forbes,* since the Great Depression, recessions in America have lasted an average of 10 months, with the longest previously being 16 months. Yet today we are more than 5 years since the end of the recession in June 2009 and the effective unemployment rate, as explained above, is really above 10 percent.

There has been no shortage of money thrown at the problem by the Obama administration. There has been the $1.2 Trillion "Stimulus" package of 2009, which failed to stimulate the job market. Then there was the "Cash for Clunkers" stimulus of early 2010, which paid back the auto industry for their support of President Obama, but again failed to stimulate the economy. Then President Obama declared the "Recovery Summer" in June of 2010, but the job market continued to decline. Even when some of the economic benchmarks began to improve, the job market lagged behind (Figure 3). Economists began referring to this as a "jobless recovery".

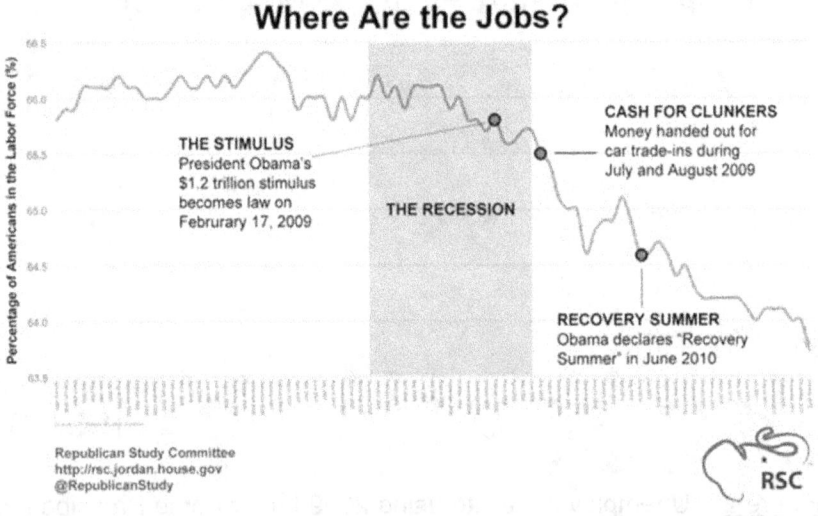

Figure 3 – The declining labor participation despite government stimulus programs.

The Impact of ObamaCare on Jobs

How do we explain this "jobless recovery"? Typically, the deeper the recession, the more robust the recovery. But not so this time. There may be disagreement among economists on the nuances of this slow recovery, but there is little disagreement that ObamaCare has been one of the important factors.

This legislation was passed on March 23, 2010, just nine months after the end of the recession in June 2009. Employers knew it was coming since it was debated for all of 2009 and early 2010. Many stood on the sidelines, waiting to see the final version of the law to calculate its impact on their business. It now seems they were wise to wait because the impact has been significant.

The Employer Mandate

The Affordable Care Act requires all employers with fifty or more full-time equivalent employees to provide health insurance for these employees or pay a fine. Full-time equivalence (FTE) is defined as 30 or more hours/week (actually 120 hours/month). If you fail to provide health insurance that qualifies under the ObamaCare standards, you must pay a fine of $2000/employee over the first 30 employees.

For example, if you have 80 FTE employees and you fail to provide their health insurance, you will be fined $2000 x 50 (80 − 30) = $100,000. If you provide health insurance, but it is too expensive (exceeds 9.5% of the employee's income) and that employee purchases insurance separately on the health insurance exchanges, you will be fined $3000/employee.

These rules were supposed to go into effect on January 1, 2014, but President Obama delayed the Employer Mandate, for political reasons, until January 1, 2015, for all employers. On January 1, 2015, employers with 100 or more employees must cover 70% of their full-time employees' healthcare coverage and 95% by 2016. Employers with 50-99 employees must cover at least 95% of employees' coverage by 2016. The employer must choose a look-back period of at least 3 months and at most 12 months. If an employee averages 30 or more hours per week in that look-back period, the employee is considered full-time.

As an employer, the way to avoid these increased costs is to reduce as many workers to part-time status (less than 30 hours/week) as possible and avoid hiring more than 49 full-time workers. This is exactly what has happened. To study the impact of ObamaCare on the workforce, The Heritage Foundation's Filip Jolevski and James Sherk looked at the average hours worked per week by lower and higher-wage workers.

Jolevski and Sherk studied the Current Population Study and found that during the recession, most earning quintiles had a net loss of full-time jobs, and the bottom three earning quintiles had a loss of average hours worked per week. But, after the recession ended in 2009, the top four quintiles began to recover full-time jobs and average hours worked per week increased substantially, whereas the bottom quintile did not recover. The ACA passed in 2010.

Since the marginal cost of providing health insurance for low-income workers is higher than for high-income workers, you would expect low-income workers to have their hours reduced to below 30 more often. This is good for employers who lower their costs for providing health insurance.

But, in a perverse way, it is also good for workers. ObamaCare creates incentives for low-income workers to purchase their health insurance on the insurance exchanges, rather than get it from their employers. The employers save money from this arrangement, but the workers can also save money.

If the employer provides insurance to the employee, but not his family, then the employee must purchase health insurance for his family. But the rules of ObamaCare prohibit the employee from purchasing the insurance for his family on the exchanges – where he would be eligible for tax credits. He must purchase the insurance from his employer's insurance provider.

However, if the employer drops his hours below 30 and he is no longer eligible for employer-provided insurance, he is now eligible to purchase his insurance for his whole family on the insurance exchanges – and get a subsidy! Therefore, he benefits from his employer dropping his health insurance. As a result of these perverse incentives, the number of part-time employees is rising. Many people are getting two or more part-time jobs.

Casey Mulligan, economist at The University of Chicago, has studied this provision of the ACA and calls this *"an implicit tax on full-time employment"*. The tax can be as much as $10,000 per year. Furthermore, this tax reduces incentives to work full-time since workers risk losing these subsidies if they take a full-time job that offers employer-provided insurance.

Here's how it works. If you are an employee considering two offers – one full-time with higher wages and healthcare benefits and one part-time with lower wages and no healthcare benefits – which one do you take? At first glance, you might think the full-time job is better – traditionally it has been.

But now you must consider the cost of providing healthcare insurance for your whole family. The full-time job provides insurance for you, but not your family. You must pay for their health insurance out of your own pocket and you are not eligible for any subsidies on the exchanges. The part-time job, however, may pay less but it offers you the chance to purchase healthcare insurance for the whole family on the exchanges *with a subsidy*.

When taxes and health expenses are accounted for, Mulligan concludes that the part-time employee would earn more each year than the full-time employee would.

Here's the scenario:

- Full-time work (at 40 hrs/week) would cost the employee $100 each week in commuting and childcare expenses and offers total gross compensation (which includes salary was well as benefits) of $52,000.

- The part-time position (at 29 hrs/week) would cost $75 in commuting and childcare expenses and offers gross compensation of $37,700.
- The full-time position provides employer-sponsored health insurance (meaning the employee would pay part of his health costs and would not be eligible for subsidies if he went to the exchanges), while the part-time position would make the employee eligible for federal subsidies.

After accounting for the costs of each health insurance option, Mulligan calculates the employee would actually earn more in the part-time position - earning $28,854 in the part-time position but just $27,021 in the full-time job. Mulligan's research estimates ObamaCare will ultimately reduce employment and hours worked by over 3 percent – the equivalent, he explains, of 4 million full-time workers. He expects this will lower our Gross Domestic Product (GDP) by 2 percent annually.

In other words, *ObamaCare is a powerful incentive for low-income workers to work less – and depend more on the government!*

The Federal Reserve Bank Surveys

In an effort to evaluate the impact of ObamaCare on the job market, three Federal Reserve Banks – in Philadelphia, New York, and Atlanta – conducted surveys of area businesses. Their findings were released in August 2014 and revealed the following:

Federal Reserve Bank of Philadelphia
- *18.2% of employers say they cut workers versus 3.0% who hired more.*
- *18.2% say the proportion of part-time workers is higher versus 1.5% who say it is lower.*
- *13.7% reported more outsourcing to other firms versus 3% with less outsourcing.*

Federal Reserve Bank of New York

- *21% of manufacturers say they are reducing employment, while 3% are increasing their workforce.*
- *In the business leaders survey on the same issue the responses were 16.9% versus 1.6%.*
- *Among manufacturers, 19.3% say they are increasing the proportion of part-time work, while 3.5% say they are reducing it.*
- *In the business leaders survey on the same question the numbers are 20.2% versus 4.8%.*

Federal Reserve Bank of Atlanta

- *34% of businesses planned to hire more part-time workers than in the past, mostly because of a rise in the relative costs of their full-time colleagues.*

In specific questioning about the impact of ObamaCare, the New York survey is especially informative:

- More than one third of manufacturers say that ObamaCare is increasing costs "a lot" this year and more than half say the health law will increase costs "a lot" next year.
- Among New York business leaders, more than one in four say ObamaCare is increasing costs "a lot" this year and more than one third predict substantial cost increases next year.

Economist John C. Goodman says, *"The new health law is discouraging a significant number of firms from hiring and is also pushing workers into part-time, rather than full time jobs."* He also points out the academic works of other economists such as Casey Mulligan, The University of Chicago, and Greg Mankiw of Harvard University.

Mulligan has calculated the marginal costs of working due to the perverse incentives of ObamaCare and concluded that ObamaCare lowers the return from working by 10%. In other words, disincentives in ObamaCare keep people from going back to work. Mankiw explains this negative effect on workers results in a loss to the economy on the order of 5% of GDP – or more than $800 Billion a year at current prices. Fewer workers means less produced. The indirect cost to the economy, as a result, equals more than $8,000 per household per year.

Three Negative Impacts

Avik Roy, healthcare policy analyst for *Forbes,* believes there are at least three negative impacts of ObamaCare on the job market:

1. ObamaCare is one of the largest tax increases in U.S. history

ObamaCare increases taxes by more than $1.2 Trillion over the next decade, making it one of the largest tax increases in U.S. history. The largest of these tax increases is the 40% tax imposed on "Cadillac plans" beginning in 2018. There is also the 3.8% surtax on investment income for high earners and businesses filing as individuals; a 0.9% increase in the Medicare payroll tax for high earners; the individual mandate tax imposed on everyone who fails to purchase health insurance; the employer mandate tax (mentioned above); and the excise taxes on health insurance premiums ($63/premium/year), medical devices, and pharmaceuticals.

Most perverse for the job market is the tax on investment income as it affects small businesses. According to Ernst & Young, 54 percent of the private-sector workforce is subject to the individual income tax rate. While not all of those businesses earn enough income to be affected by the ObamaCare tax, affected businesses will have to make up the difference by either hiring fewer workers, or charging higher prices for their goods and services, or both.

2. *ObamaCare increases the cost of employing workers*

As detailed above, the employer mandate requires employers to provide health insurance or pay substantial taxes. The employer mandate is a strong incentive for small businesses to keep their work force under 50 full-time employees and to move full-time employees to part-time status.

For those employers who do provide heath insurance to their workers, the costs of that health insurance are going up because of ObamaCare. The required "essential health benefits" compels employers to purchase insurance plans that provide benefits many of them do not need, yet they must pay for them nevertheless. This increases the cost for everyone. As labor costs go up, employers have less money to employ more workers.

3. *ObamaCare's exchange subsidies encourage many workers to drop out*

Roy is referring here to the work of Casey Mulligan again. He finds that ObamaCare's subsidies are *"roughly equivalent to doubling both employer and employee payroll tax rates for half of the population."* In other words, the half of the population that is eligible for ObamaCare subsidies.

Some supporters of ObamaCare have pointed to the experience of Massachusetts under Romneycare – where labor force participation was not substantially affected – as proof that ObamaCare will do fine on this score. But Mulligan estimates that *"the ACA will increase the national average marginal labor income tax rate about fourteen times more than the 2006 'Romneycare' health reform law increased the Massachusetts average rate."*

The Walmart Response

Walmart is the nation's largest private employer with about 1.4 million employees. In October 2014 they are dropping health benefits for some 30,000 workers, or about 5% of its part-time workforce. Earlier in 2011, health-plan eligibility triage had removed tens of thousands of Walmart workers from the company balance sheets.

Walmart cites its inability to manage higher-than-anticipated health expenses. This follows similar moves by competitors Target, Home Depot, and Trader Joe's. Walmart said it would drop coverage beginning January 1, 2015 for existing workers who were grandfathered into the company's heath plan. Now, only those part-timers working 30 to 34 hours a week will qualify for the company's health coverage. (ObamaCare defines these "part-timers" as full-time and compels the company to provide their health insurance or pay a tax.)

Walmart is also raising premiums for all workers in 2015. About 40% of enrolled workers are on its least expensive and most popular plan. They will now pay $21.90 per two-week pay period, a 20% increase beginning January 1. Across all three plans, Walmart said it estimates workers will pay an additional $10/pay period. The average Walmart hourly worker earns $11.81 per hour.

Ironically, Walmart was a big supporter of ObamaCare in its early days before passage. But now they see the writing on the wall. *"We can't take our eyes off costs,"* said Sally Welborn, senior vice president of global benefits at Walmart. Walmart forecasts that its health-care costs will rise by $500 million *more than it had expected* in the year ending January 31, 2015.

This move by the nation's largest employer confirms the impressions given in the Federal Reserve Banks Survey mentioned above. Employers can't ignore the impact of ObamaCare on their employee benefit costs. Shelly Banjo, Anna Wilde Mathews, and Theo Francis, writing in the *Wall Street Journal,* document the same changes are happening at many other businesses.

"Many businesses are continuing to shift more costs to workers. Phoenix-based technology distributor Avnet Inc., for example, is paring back its traditional plans in favor of high-deductible options. Other companies are reducing coverage for spouses, according to consultants at Towers Watson & Co. Still others are going further,

ending their traditional coverage for employees who will instead get a fixed sum of money to buy their own insurance on private exchanges. Aon PLC's Aon Hewitt is set to announce that enrollment in its exchange will grow to around 850,000 workers and dependents next year as another 15 employers sign up."

They go on to point out that private-sector employers spent $446 billion on health insurance premiums in 2012, the most recent year for which the federal Medicare agency has published figures, and they were expected to pay $483 Billion this year, up 22% from 2007. Households spent $284 Billion on premiums in 2012. They are expected to spend slightly less this year to $282 billion, but it is still up 20% from 2007.

The "Cadillac Tax" Impact

The 40% tax on "Cadillac plans" doesn't begin until 2018 but the impact is being felt already. A survey released in August by the National Business Group on Health found that, to minimize the impact of the tax, 57% of employers were planning to implement or expand high-deductible plans, while 42% were boosting employees' cost-sharing. In other words, employers are passing more of the cost of these plans onto their employees.

Randall Abbott, a senior consultant at Towers Watson, says employers are extremely concerned about this tax and cites moves to high-deductible plans by FedEx Corp. and JetBlue as evidence. Avnet, the technology distributor, also added two new high-deductible plans this year. All of Avnet's plans next year will have at least a $1500 deductible for a single worker, although the company will also contribute as much as $500 to employees' HSA accounts. A spokesman for the company estimated the tax would cost them $1.4 million in 2018 unless they made changes.

The Impact on Innovation

The impact of ObamaCare on the job market was easily predictable. When you punish employers for increasing their labor force beyond 50 full-time employees or beyond 30-hour workweeks, you can expect them to stop hiring or to adjust to more part-time workers. What is less predictable is the impact of the law on innovation.

It is well known that the United States leads the world in medical innovations. No one develops more break-through drug treatments, surgical procedures, medical devices, patents, diagnostic improvements, and other new ideas in medical treatment.

Scott W. Atlas, a physician and senior fellow at Stanford University's Hoover Institution, says among the many unintended consequences of the Affordable Care Act, the least noticed is its threat to innovation. Most of the funding for that innovation – about 71% of U.S. research and development investment – comes from private industry. A recent survey by R & D Magazine of industry leaders in 63 countries ranked the U.S. number one in the world for health-care innovation.

However, Atlas says that situation is changing. According to R & D Magazine and the research firm Battelle, growth of R & D spending in the U.S from 2012 to 2014 averaged just 2.1%, down from an average of 6% over the previous 15 years. In that same 15-year period, Malaysia, Thailand, Singapore, South Korea, India, and the European Union saw faster R & D spending growth than the U.S. China's grew on average 22% per year.

What accounts for these changes? To be sure, the slowdown reflects the recession of 2008/2009. But the recession affected not only the U.S. but also the whole world, including the countries mentioned above. It is clear there is more to this picture than the economic slowdown.

The economy's weakness has been exacerbated by the negative impact of new taxes and regulations under ObamaCare. According to Congressional Budget Office (CBO) estimates, the new healthcare law will levy more than $500 billion in new taxes over its first 10 years to help pay for insurance subsidies and Medicaid expansion. These new taxes include significant levies on key healthcare industries, such as manufacturers of medical devices and drugs, and their investors.

To adjust to these changes, both small and large U.S. healthcare technology companies are moving R & D centers and jobs overseas. Atlas says the CEO of one of the largest healthcare companies in America recently told him that the device tax his company paid in 2013 exceeded his company's entire R & D budget.

A long list of companies, including Boston Scientific, Stryker (a large orthopedic equipment company), and Cook Medical have announced job cuts and plans to open new centers for R & D, manufacturing and clinical trials overseas.

This alarming trend is aggravated by delays in approval of new medical technology by the Food and Drug Administration (FDA). According to a 2010 survey of more than 200 medical-device companies by medical professor and entrepreneur Josh Makower and his colleagues at Stanford University, delays of approvals for new medical devices are now far longer in the U.S. than in many other developed countries.

In the European Union it takes on average 7 months to gain approval for low to moderate-risk devices. In the U.S., FDA approval for similar devices takes on average 31 months. The impact of these delays on a manufacturer amounts to millions of dollars of lost revenue and may be the difference between profitability and loss.

How is this affecting medical innovation in the U.S.?

The 2011 Price-Waterhouse-Coopers Medical Technology Innovation Scorecard found the "the gap between innovation leaders and emerging economies is rapidly narrowing." Although the United States is expected to hold its lead, the country will continue to lose ground during the next decade. Countries such as China, India, and Brazil are expected to experience the strongest gains during the next ten years.

In a related development, since the signing of the ACA in 2010, private-equity investment in new U.S. healthcare startups has also diminished. Annual capital investment has decreased to $41 billion in 2013 from $61 billion in 2011, according to the accounting and audit firm McGladrey, LLP. Also, the Silicon Valley-based law firm Wilson Sonsini Goodrich and Rosati reported in its semiannual Life Sciences Reports, decreases from the first half of 2010 through the second half of 2013 in deal closings and capital raised for startups in biopharmaceuticals, medical devices and equipment, and diagnostics, with only a slight uptick in health-information systems investment.

Silicon Valley is the heart of the venture capital industry and the home to many of our best companies for development of new medical technology.

Atlas is also concerned about the "brain drain" effect of this exodus of medical technology. He says many of the best and brightest who come to the U.S. to study science, technology, engineering and math – the STEM subjects that are so crucial to innovation – are choosing to return to their home countries upon graduation. In 2008, a survey conducted by Vivek Wadhwa and his team of researchers at Duke, Harvard and the University of California, found that only 6% of Indian, 10% of Chinese, and 15 % of European students expected to make America their permanent home.

While this survey predates the passage of ObamaCare, the trend has only been exacerbated by the new healthcare law. He also cites Congress for their slowness to increase limits on H-1B visas for high skill foreign workers. But even if Congress were to act now, the decline in R & D spending is unlikely to convince these students to remain in the United States when there are more jobs available in their home countries.

What is the solution? The repeal of ObamaCare would go a long way toward solving this problem. In the absence of full repeal, Atlas has several suggestions:

- Repeal the ACA's $29 Billion medical device tax
- Repeal the ACA's $80 Billion tax on brand-name drugs
- Change the tax code to add incentives for investment in early stage medical technology and life-science companies

- Add incentives for philanthropic gifts to academic institutions that promote technology entrepreneurs
- Simplify the process of approval of new medical devices and pharmaceuticals

In summary of this chapter, ObamaCare is having adverse impacts on the job market and the growth of medical technology companies at a time in our history when more people have fallen out of the labor force than at any time in the last 36 years. Despite President Obama's professed interest in improving our economy and creating more jobs, his policies, especially ObamaCare, are the root cause of our continued "jobless recovery".

11

ObamaCare and Income Inequality

"A dangerous and growing inequality . . . has jeopardized middle-class America's basic bargain that if you work hard, you have a chance to get ahead."
President Barack Obama - 12/4/13

The American dream is dying. According to the Public Religion Research Institute poll in September, 2014, merely 42% of Americans still believe in the American dream. If true, then only a minority of Americans now believe that "if you work hard, you'll get ahead." The poll says the steepest declines in belief in the last two years were among people under age 30 (down 16 percentage points), women (down 14 percentage points) and Democrats (down 17 percentage points).

Stop and think about that. That means the same people (in demographic terms) that elected President Obama in large numbers are the most disillusioned after six years of his presidency. But rather than give up on him, they re-elected him for another four years.

The Wall Street Journal editorial board calls President Obama *"the best President for slow growth and inequality in modern history, as new economic surveys show."* They cite the Census Bureau's annual poverty and income survey released in October 2014. Real U.S. median household income – or the wages earned in the middle of the wage distribution – was $51,939, a 0.3% increase over 2012. But the 2013 figure is still 3.9% lower than the median income when the recession ended in 2009, and 7.9% lower than the median in 2007 (Figure 1).

Therefore, despite the fact that the recession ended over 5 years ago, the median income is lower now than its low point during the recession.

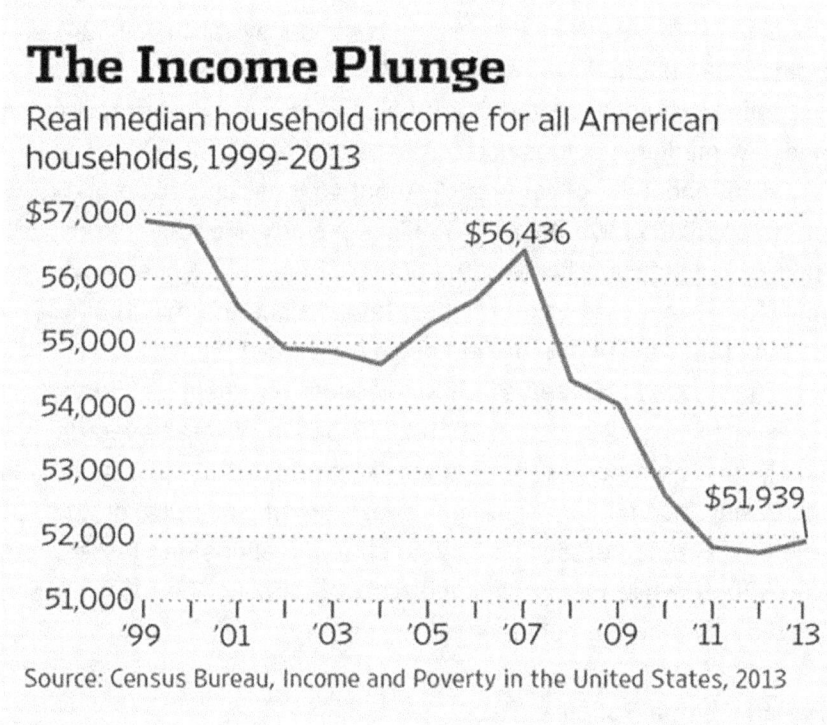

The Income Plunge

Real median household income for all American households, 1999-2013

Source: Census Bureau, Income and Poverty in the United States, 2013

Figure 1 – Real median household income 1999 – 2013

Liberals will sometimes try to argue that the median household income has been falling steadily since the height of the dot-com bubble in 1999. But Figure 1 makes it clear that there was a resurgence beginning in 2003 after the passage of the Bush tax cuts on capital income and marginal income-tax rates. Incomes rose for three straight years to a 2007 level of $56,436. The bottom fell out with the 2008 financial panic and recession that followed.

That was to be expected given the state of the economy. But what was not expected was that incomes did not rebound with the recovery as they have in every other expansion. Only in 2013 do we begin to see a rise, just barely, five long years into the recovery that started in June 2009.

What's more, the slight increase was only seen in 14 states concentrated in metro areas like Washington-Arlington-Alexandria (median: $90,149), San Francisco-Oakland-Hayward ($79,624) and Boston-Cambridge-Newton ($72,907). Wyoming was the lone state exception, which benefited from the oil and gas fracking revolution and saw median incomes rise 5.7%.

What about the poverty rate? About 45.3 million people or 14.5% of the population live below the official poverty line, down from 15% in 2012 but statistically the same number of people. Poverty over the prior four years rose to the highest levels since the mid-1960s. The poverty rate was 14.3% in 2009 and 12.5% in 2007.

The Federal Reserve also released its triennial Survey of Consumer Finances for the 2010-2013 period. Overall average real family income rose 4%, but median income fell 5%, consistent with increasing income concentration. Those Americans between the 40th and 90th income percentiles saw no changes after steep losses from 2007-2010, while median income rose 2% among the top 10% and fell 5.5% among the bottom 40%.

Failed Obama Policies

What's remarkable about these numbers is that they are happening at a time when President Obama consistently rails against income inequality and has focused his policies on reducing that inequality throughout his presidency. His stimulus package of 2009-2010 mainly provided transfer payments like Medicaid and unemployment benefits. Unemployment benefits were increased from 26 weeks when Obama took office to a staggering 99 weeks, nearly two full years.

He also expanded the number of Americans on food stamps to record numbers and increased the number of people receiving disability payments. He has raised taxes on the rich so they *"will pay their fair share"* even though they were already paying the lion's share of income taxes before. Nearly half of all Americans pay no income taxes at all.

Minimum Wage Increases

His latest gambit is raising the minimum wage to $10.10/hour. But the Democratic Congress already raised the minimum wage in three stages to $7.25/hour in 2009 from $5.15/hour in 2007. If raising the minimum wage is so beneficial to the American worker, where is the evidence? In fact, the Congressional Budget Office has estimated a raise of the minimum wage to $10.10/hour would cost workers 500,000 jobs.

The Wall Street Journal editorial board says the Census data show *that every income group that was supposed to benefit from the higher wages is worse off than before the minimum wage was increased.* This is because the benefits of mandated wage increases for some workers are dwarfed by the overall negative economic trends of slower growth and reduced opportunity.

Research by Stanford University economist Thomas Macurdy backs this up. He has studied the impact of the 1996 increase of the minimum wage from $4.25/hr. to $5.15/hr. and found unintended consequences. His peer-reviewed study is soon to be published in the Journal of Political Economy. The results show the failure of minimum-wage hikes as an antipoverty policy.

Most Americans favor minimum-wage increases because they believe it helps poor workers support their families. But Macurdy says that only about 5% of families supported by minimum-wage jobs have children. It is well known that minimum-wage increases cause many workers to lose their jobs. But advocates argue that the number of workers who gain far exceeds those who lose. Macurdy's research challenges this assertion.

The important issue to consider is where the money comes from. Any higher wage must be paid by someone. A higher wage is paid by the consumer of the product that company produces. But will low-income families earn more from an increase in the minimum wage than they will pay as consumers of the now higher-priced goods. Macurdy's research strongly suggests they won't.

To understand why we must first recognize that minimum-wage workers are typically not in low-income families; instead they are dispersed evenly among families rich, middle-class and poor. About one in five families in the bottom fifth of the income distribution had a minimum-wage worker affected by the 1996 increase, the same share as for families in the top fifth.

Virtually as much of the additional earnings of minimum-wage workers went to the highest-income families as to the lowest. Moreover, only about $1 in $5 of the addition went to families with children supported by low-wage earnings.

Second, we must examine who actually bears the burden of higher labor costs that are passed on through higher prices of goods and services. Macurdy's analysis, using the Bureau of Labor Statistics' Consumer Expenditure Survey, showed that the 1996 minimum-wage hike raised prices on a broad variety of goods and services. Food purchased outside of the home bore the largest share of the increased consumption costs, accounting for 21%; the next highest shares were around 10% for retail services, groceries and household personal services.

The higher prices actually resembled a regressive value-added, or sales, tax, with *rates rising the lower a family's income.* Unlike normal tax policy, which strives to impact low-income families less than high-income families, this policy harms the poor more. Macurdy summarizes:

*"My analysis concludes that more poor families were losers than winners from the 1996 hike in the minimum wage. Nearly one in five low-income families benefited, but **all low-income families paid for the increase through higher prices.***

Consider a McDonald's restaurant, often cited as ground zero in minimum wage debates. To cover costs of a mandated increase in the earnings of McDonald's lowest-paid workers, customers pay more for the company's food. The distributional question becomes: Which group comes from the least well-off families: McDonald's customers or its lowest-paid workers? Economy-wide evidence show that the customers disproportionately come from low-income families."

Employers, like CKE Restaurants, can attest to the real impact of raising the minimum wage. Andy Puzder, CEO of this chain of restaurants, explains:

"Our typical franchised restaurant employs 25 people and earns about $100,000 a year in pretax profit – about 8% of the restaurant's $1.2 million annual sales. Our general managers, often also the store owners, are responsible for the success or failure of the business. They manage the employees and are in charge of a million-dollar facility. General managers are responsible for at least 25% of store profits. The other 24 employees are responsible for the remaining 75%, which comes to about $3,125 an employee. That is a generous estimate, as entry-level employees likely contribute less than their more experienced colleagues.

If minimum-wage crewmembers working 25 hours a week received a 40% raise, they would earn an additional $3,705 a year. That is $580 more than what the employee contributors to the restaurant's profits. The point is simple: The feds can mandate a higher wage, but some jobs don't produce enough economic value to bear the increase. If government could transform unskilled entry-level positions into middle-income jobs, the Soviet Union would be today's dominant world economy. Spain and Greece would be thriving."

Puzder goes on to explain that the only way a business like his can adapt to a mandated raise in the minimum wage is to cut jobs and rely more on technology. These changes are already happening in banks, gas stations, grocery stores, airports, and restaurants.

Less than three weeks after Puzder's Op-Ed in *The Wall Street Journal* was published, McDonald's reported a 30% decline in quarterly profits on a 5% drop in revenues. The earnings report revealed the company plans to respond to the pressure to increase minimum wages by automation.

By the third quarter of next year, McDonald's plans to introduce new technology in some markets *"to make it easier for customers to order and pay for food digitally and to give people the ability to customize their orders."* CEO Don Thompson said customers *"want to personalize their meals"* and *"to enjoy eating in a contemporary, inviting atmosphere. And they want choices in how they order, choices in what they order and how they're served."*

This is really an excuse to justify a reduction in the chain's global workforce, according to the Editorial board of *The Wall Street Journal*. It's also a way to send a message to franchisees about the best way to reduce their costs amid slow sales growth and pressure to increase the minimum wage.

The impact of raising the minimum wage can already be measured in the Bay Area cities of San Francisco and Oakland, California. In November, 2014, voters approved raising the minimum wage to $15/hour in San Francisco and $12.25/hour in Oakland for most businesses in the city boundaries. Now the bills to pay for these wage increases can't be paid.

Michael Saltsman, research director at the Employment Policies Institute, writes in *The Wall Street Journal* that businesses are going bankrupt and jobs are being lost. This is no surprise to labor economists. A summary of the research published last year by the Institute for the Study of Labor, and authored by University of California-Irvine economist David Neumark, found that each 10% hike in the minimum wage on the state and federal level has caused a 1% to 2% drop in youth employment. Also, researchers at the Federal Reserve Bank of Chicago found an increase in fast-food prices associated with the same wage change.

Businesses first respond to these labor-cost increases by raising prices. In Oakland, local restaurants are raising prices by as much as 20%, with the San Francisco Chronicle reporting that "some of the city's top restaurateurs fear they will lose customers to higher prices." This fear was justified since many formerly successful restaurants have gone bankrupt since the wage increase.

The Abbot's Cellar, twice selected as one of the city's top-100 restaurants, has since closed. One of the partners explained the restaurant had no ability to absorb the added cost, and neither a miraculous increase in sales volume nor higher prices were viable options. In the city's popular SoMa neighborhood, a vegetarian diner called The Source closed in January, again citing the higher minimum wage as a factor.

Back across the Bay in Oakland, the Chronicle reported that some of the city's businesses have been similarly affected. According to a board member of the Oakland Chinatown Chamber of Commerce, 10 restaurants or grocery stores opted to permanently close this year alone as a partial consequence of the wage hike. Even the Salvation Army's child-care facility is "scrambling to find ways to keep the doors open" in response to labor cost increase, according to the organization's county coordinator.

Businesses go bankrupt, jobs are lost, prices go up even in fast-food restaurants that especially cater to low-income families, and shelters for the poor like the Salvation Army struggle to survive. These are the unintended consequences of raising the minimum wage.

Yet those who advocate these policies are not convinced. Ken Jacobs, director of the University of California-Berkeley's labor-backed Center for Labor Research and Education, chalked up possible consequences of new mandates to labor-market "churn." Research that Jacobs co-authored predicted that the Bay Area hikes would be mostly cost-free. At a forum in March, 2015, where dozens of Oakland business owners worried about their viability, representatives of Lift Up Oakland – the labor union-backed coalition that advocated for the wage hike – were not in attendance.

Monetary Policy

Another factor in this perverse economic recovery has been the Obama administration monetary policy. The Federal Reserve's Quantitative Easing (QE) has been targeted at raising asset prices, such as stocks and real estate. This policy, by creating nearly negligible interest rates, has fueled growth in stocks and real estate. These assets are disproportionately owned by the affluent and not low to moderate-income workers. Those who own these assets have seen substantial gains in the market value of their assets. Conversely, those low to moderate-income workers, who own savings accounts, have seen nearly negligible returns on their investments. The result of these differences is greater income inequality.

Unfortunately, instead of learning from the mistakes of the past, liberals point to rising income inequality and call for more of the same policies that have created the currently widening income gap. By putting more emphasis on equality than on economic growth, President Obama has both reduced growth and increased inequality.

The Kaiser Family Foundation Survey

The Kaiser Family Foundation is a left-leaning think-tank concerned with healthcare in America. They reported that health insurance premiums rose by a "modest 3%" in 2013. However, even more modest was the 2.3% growth of workers' earnings last year. This tells us that healthcare costs are rising faster than wages. In fact, government data show that healthcare costs are the biggest driver of income inequality in America today.

Mark J. Warshawsky and Andrew G. Biggs, writing in *The Wall Street Journal,* analyzed this data. They say that when employers' costs for benefits like health insurance rise, they will hold back on salary increases to keep total compensation costs in check. The Bureau of Labor Statistics (BLS) confirms that's exactly what is happening. BLS data show that from June 2004 to June 2014 compensation increased by 28% while employer health insurance costs rose by 51%. Therefore, average wages grew by just 23%. But the impact is felt more severely by low to moderate-income workers.

Let's put some real numbers on the table to make it clearer. An average family health policy today costs employers nearly $12,000 per year, up from only $4,200 in 1999. That's about a 200% increase in only 15 years or nearly triple the cost in 1999. If employer health insurance premiums had not risen, average salaries today would be around $7,800 higher.

Consider a lower-income worker who makes today $30,000 per year. If he made $7,800 more that would be a 26% salary increase. By contrast, a high-income worker who today makes $250,000, would have seen his earnings rise by only 3.1% if he got the same salary increase. Therefore health costs are a bigger share of total compensation for lower-wage workers, so rising health costs impact their salaries much more. This contributes to income inequality.

The BLS National Compensation Survey confirms this is what is happening. For low-income workers, total pay and benefits rose by 41% from 1999 through 2006. But because of the high cost of healthcare benefits, their wages rose only 28%, which barely outpaces inflation. During this same period, employer costs for healthcare benefits nearly doubled from 6.5% to 12.2% of compensation.

In contrast, the BLS data show that compensation for workers earning $250,000 or more per year rose by 36% from 1999 through 2006. That's actually less than the 41% growth in compensation experienced by low-income workers over the same timeframe. But healthcare benefits costs for this group rose from 4% of compensation in 1999 to only 4.3% in 2006.

Since healthcare costs are a much smaller part of their total pay and benefits, the salaries of these high-income workers grew by 35%, a faster rate than for low-wage workers. The inequality of total compensation barely changed from 1999-2006, but rising healthcare costs held back the growth of low and middle-class earnings.

Therefore, the take-home message is this: *The more we spend on health care the greater the income inequality between low-income and high-income workers.*

The Impact of ObamaCare on Inequality

Left out of this discussion, so far, has been the role of ObamaCare in contributing to income inequality. You might assume that it has improved the situation for low to moderate-income workers since ObamaCare was designed to provide "free" health care to millions of these Americans. If nothing else, ObamaCare is really a "wealth re-distribution" vehicle that transfers wealth from high-income Americans to low-income Americans.

But it's really much more complicated than that. Chris Conover, healthcare analyst writing in *Forbes,* suggests ObamaCare may actually be making the income inequality situation worse. But first some background information is needed.

The Cost of Health Benefits

To understand the impact of ObamaCare we must first discuss the impact of healthcare benefits on workers' wages. A 2011 study released by Towers Watson states the following:

- For workers in the lowest 10% of the earnings distribution the cost to employers to provide health benefits is equivalent to a 49.5% increase in cash wages.
- For the highest income workers, the cost of this same benefit is only one seventh as large or 6.3%.

Health benefits add 50 percent to the cost of hiring low-wage workers

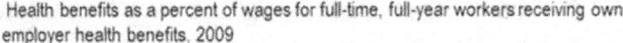

Health benefits as a percent of wages for full-time, full-year workers receiving own employer health benefits, 2009

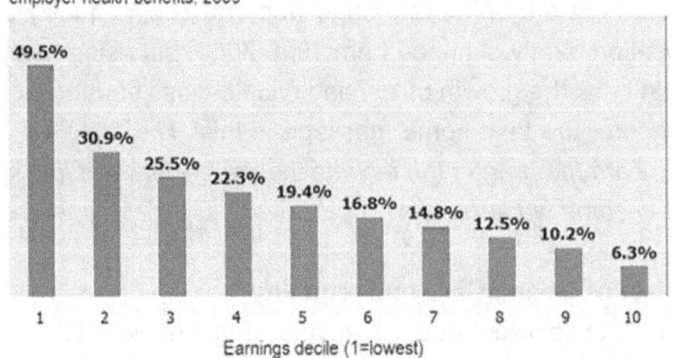

Source: Steven Nyce and Sylvester Schieber, Treating Our Ills and Killing Our Prospects. Towers Watson, August 3, 2011. http://www.towerswatson.com/en-US/Insights/IC-Types/Survey-Research-Results/2011/08/Treating-Our-Ills-and-Killing-Our-Prospects

Figure 2 – Health benefits as a percentage of wages. Health benefits represent a higher percentage of wages for low-income workers.

From the chart in Figure 2 we see how health benefits represent a much higher percentage of wages for low-income workers than those with higher incomes. That means low-wage workers are disproportionately affected by every $100 added to employer-paid health insurance premiums. The authors of the study calculated that for the lowest-paid 10% of workers, 112% of all the compensation gains between 1980-2009 were absorbed by more expensive health benefits, compared to only 8% for those in the highest decile of worker earnings.

What do these numbers really mean? They mean that those in the lowest wage group actually experienced a *negative* increase in cash compensation (their take-home wages went down). The added cost to provide health benefits ate up every penny of any increase in compensation earned – and then some!

In contrast, workers at the upper end of the earnings distribution were able to absorb the equivalent increase in employer-paid health insurance premiums while still leaving 92% of their compensation gains to be paid in the form of higher cash wages or other fringe benefits such as retirement contributions.

To be clear, the employers are compensating both groups of workers with the same increase in benefits. Both are getting healthcare benefits that cost about the same. However, because of the differences in their wages, the relative cost to the low-income worker is much higher and the net take-home wage actually goes down.

How ObamaCare Will Aggravate This Trend

Conover explains that under ObamaCare, low-wage workers who qualify for insurance exchange coverage will avoid being trapped in health plans whose ever-riding costs absorb a disproportionate share of their future compensation. But the combination of the Individual Mandate and Employer Mandate will force low-wage workers in larger firms not only to have more expensive coverage than they did in the past, but also to pay for it in the form of foregone wages.

In other words, if you work for a large company that must provide health benefits (due to the Employer Mandate) you will be ineligible for the taxpayer subsidies that are only available on the insurance exchanges. The value of these subsidies can be as much as $18,000 a year for the lowest-income families. Not only will you lose these subsidies, but your wages will be blunted by the employer's high cost of keeping you on the company health insurance plan. Both you and your employer will be adversely impacted.

Figure 3 shows how low-wage workers bear a disproportionately higher cost of health benefits due to ObamaCare. For the lowest decile, the cost of health benefits imposed by ObamaCare is 134.4% of compensation gains – or a net *negative* gain. For the highest decile, the cost of health benefits imposed by ObamaCare is only 20.3% of compensation gains – they still see a 79.7% gain in real take-home wages.

Low-wage workers in employer-based plans will bear the brunt of burdens imposed by the Affordable Care Act

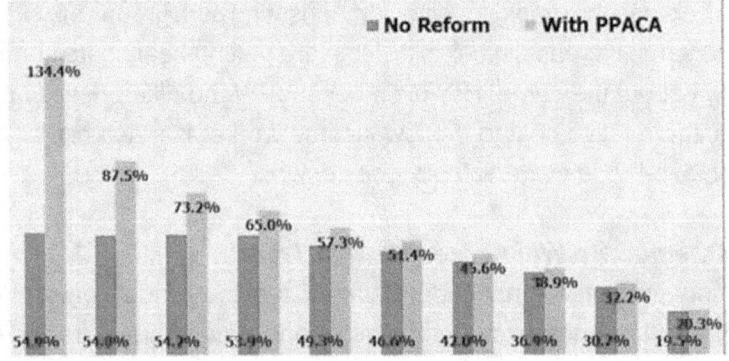

Share of compensation gains provided in the form of more expensive health benefits paid by employers for full-year workers assuming current inflation rates, 2015-2030

Source: Steven Nyce and Sylvester Schieber, Treating Our Ills and Killing Our Prospects. Towers Watson, August 3, 2011. http://www.towerswatson.com/en-US/Insights/IC-Types/Survey-Research-Results/2011/08/Treating-Our-Ills-and-Killing-Our-Prospects

<u>Figure 3</u> - The impact of ObamaCare on wages. Low-wage workers bear a higher proportion of the cost of health benefits.

The cost of health benefits, admittedly, will always be higher for low-wage workers than high-wage workers. But Figure 3 shows how ObamaCare has greatly exaggerated this difference – and therefore contributed adversely to income inequality. Conover summarizes:

"By increasing the cost of coverage through mandated benefits that low-wage workers may not necessarily need or want, ObamaCare virtually ensures that the lowest wage workers will continue to experience negative cash wage growth through the year 2030."

This discussion has revealed the adverse impacts of ObamaCare on the wages of workers. But there are also the perverse incentives ObamaCare will create in the real world as employers and workers strive to adjust to these changes imposed by the law.

Millions of workers will move to part-time status to avoid the disparities in compensation we have just discussed. As outlined in the previous chapter, workers may benefit greatly by holding down two part-time jobs rather than one full-time job. In fact, as the analysis of Casey Mulligan revealed in Chapter 10, they may be better off with even *one* part-time job. Here is another analysis by Mulligan:

"The ACA's long-term impact will include about 3% less weekly employment, 3% fewer aggregate work hours, 2% less GDP and 2% less labor income. These effects will be visible and obvious by 2017, if not before. The employment and hours estimates are based on the combined amount of the law's new taxes and disincentives and on historical research on the aggregate effects of each dollar of Taxation. The GDP and income estimates reflect lower amounts of labor as well as the law's effects on the productivity of each hour of labor."

Mulligan is predicting the following:

- 3% less weekly employment
- 3% fewer work hours
- 2% less GDP (Gross National Product)
- 2% less labor income

You don't have to be an economist to understand that *fewer workers, working less, producing less, and earning less is no way to solve the income inequality problem - nor improve the economy or the strength of our nation.*

Conover emphasizes the importance of getting rid of the Individual and Employer Mandates to avoid these perverse outcomes. He recommends all Americans receive standardized tax credits, much like the system in Switzerland. We'll discuss in more detail alternative proposals for ObamaCare, as they have evolved since my first book on this subject, in the next chapter.

12

Alternatives That Work

"The Affordable Care Act is here to stay."
President Barack Obama
Rose Garden ceremony - 4/1/14

Things are not always what they seem. Despite President Obama's declaration that *"The Affordable Care Act is here to stay,"* there is ample evidence to the contrary. Polls continue to show a majority of Americans are opposed to the law despite Democratic claims that people would like it the more they got to know it.

But people don't want to go back to the previous status quo, either. Recent polls repeatedly show that a clear majority of voters want a better alternative if ObamaCare is to be replaced. When given a choice between (a) keeping or "fixing" ObamaCare and (b) repealing it in the absence of an alternative, repeal splits the electorate evenly. When they are given a choice between (a) keeping or "fixing" ObamaCare and (b) repealing it in the context of a conservative alternative, repeal becomes a nearly 2 to 1 winner.

This presents Republicans with a clear mandate – *replace ObamaCare with a better alternative.*

To be sure, a better alternative must appeal to both sides of the aisle, Democrats as well as Republicans. It is a major flaw of ObamaCare that it was passed without a single Republican vote. No other entitlement lacked bipartisan support and no other entitlement is less popular than ObamaCare. In reality, this may not be possible before a change of the presidency, but Republicans must show they've got the right ideas and they'll implement them if the voters give them the chance.

There has been no shortage of Republican ideas. Several bills have been introduced in Congress dating back to 2009 before the passage of ObamaCare. The Patient Choice Act was introduced by Congressman Paul Ryan (R – WI) on May 20, 2009. Other bills include The Empowering Patients First Act introduced by Congressman Tom Price (R – GA) in 2009 and The American Health Care Reform Act introduced by Congressman Phil Roe (R – TN) in 2013.

In 2014, Senator Tom Coburn (R – OK) introduced a bill in the Senate similar to the Ryan bill in the House. Recently his bill was re-introduced with some changes and co-sponsored by Sen. Burr (R – NC) and Sen. Hatch (R – UT). It is now known as The Patient CARE Act.

Plans Introduced in Congress

For a review of these plans I am reprinting here my remarks from my first book, *The ObamaCare Train Wreck,* which summarizes each plan:

"The Empowering Patients First Act (HR 2300) introduced by Rep. Tom Price (GA) calls for tax credits and refundable tax credits with means testing, as well as tax deductions for all Americans who purchase health insurance. Tax credits return money to low income Americans who pay taxes. Refundable tax credits are payments to low income Americans who pay no taxes at all. Both lower the cost of purchasing health insurance for low-income families and increase the rolls of the insured – the principal purpose of ObamaCare.

Tax deductions, on the other hand, level the playing field for all those who purchase their insurance on the individual market. Currently, those Americans who receive their insurance through their employer pay no taxes on this benefit. Those who purchase their insurance on the individual market must do so with after-tax dollars. This system has existed since the post- World War II days when wage controls prohibited companies from increasing wages to attract new workers. Health insurance and other benefits were added as an incentive for new workers, but these benefits were never taxed. This system still exists today.

The American Health Care Reform Act (HR 3121) introduced by Rep. Phil Roe (TN) does not include tax credits but does provide for a $7,500 tax deduction for individuals and $20,000 for families. Families can keep the full deduction even if they spend less (to eliminate the incentive to spend more on health insurance) and invest the difference in a HSA.

The Patient CARE Act introduced in the Senate seeks to gradually eliminate the tax discrepancy between employer and individual plans by imposing a tax exclusion cap of 65% on the average cost of employer provided plans. Avik Roy of Forbes calls this plan "the most credible plan yet". He states it was scored by former CBO director Douglas Holtz-Eakin's Center for Health and Economy and they report this plan would reduce the deficit by $1.5 Trillion dollars over ten years. Although some have criticized this plan as a "big tax hike", Roy points out that it would lower the deficit by $416 Billion over ten years even without the tax increase.

This plan seems to be gaining traction. It was hailed by Yuval Levin and Ramesh Ponnuru of National Review in an article called "At Last, the Replacement". They call it "the first one that is also competitive with ObamaCare in the number of people it would cover and would not cause those who have employer-provided insurance to lose it." Studies by the University of Minnesota's Center for Health and Economy suggest it would actually enable about 2 million more people to get coverage over the coming decade than ObamaCare would, at much lower cost.

Liberals have tried to portray it as a tax hike because it caps the tax exclusion on employer-provided plans. However, with its repeal of ObamaCare's tax increases, Levin and Ponnuru point out it would actually amount to a large tax cut when compared to ObamaCare. Furthermore, the authors of the bill have said that if the cap ends up collecting revenue that exceeds the cost of the new credit, they would raise that cap accordingly.

Other liberals have tried to pretend this bill is so similar to ObamaCare that it actually is an endorsement of ObamaCare - they call "ObamaCare Lite". They point to the "narrow networks" of both plans, disregarding the fact that ObamaCare offers no choice in these networks, which are necessary as the only way insurance providers can offer cheaper plans. Both plans offer insurance on your parents' plan up to age 26, both offer caps on the tax exclusion for employer-provided coverage, and both provide subsidies for purchasing insurance on the individual market.

But ObamaCare is more coercive, forcing great numbers of people into heavily regulated exchanges. The Republican alternative has no exchanges. It cap is only to restrain the incentive for ever-higher health-care spending and to fund the new tax credit. Therefore, it encourages and enables people to become more discerning consumers of health insurance. The ObamaCare subsidies are needed to overcome the disincentives of purchasing coverage that the law's burdensome rules creates. In the Republican proposal they are intended to enable people to enter a competitive insurance marketplace as consumers with real purchasing power.

All of this highlights the stark differences in liberal and conservative approaches to health care reform. Liberals approach the issue from the paternalistic view that they have figured out what's best for the country and the people and they must coerce compliance with their ideas by imposing penalties for non-compliance and off-setting the costs and risks with taxpayer dollars.

Levin and Ponnuru put it this way, "It would have been politically unviable for the government to simply take over health insurance and directly apply the vision of experts. But the law is moved by the same basic logic as a single-payer system: We have the answer and need to impose it on everyone from above."

Conservatives, on the other hand, begin with the premise that they do not have all the answers but that the most likely way to achieve success is through a genuinely competitive market in which insurers may offer a range of options and consumers have the resources and the freedom to choose among them. Such a system creates powerful incentives for everyone to seek the proper balance through constant innovation and improvement.

There is one similarity between the two systems that could be improved; both have means-tested subsidies that phase out as income rises. This causes a disincentive to work harder and make more money only to see the loss of the insurance subsidy. A better way would be to have a flat, universal benefit that eliminates such a disincentive to climb the economic ladder."

This completes the summary of those proposals already introduced in Congress. Figure 1 provides a side-by-side comparison of The Patient CARE Act with ObamaCare. Since the publication of my first book, other proposals have been suggested in the media that will be discussed now.

The Goodman Proposal

Economist and healthcare analyst John C. Goodman has unveiled his proposals. Writing in *National Review*, he outlines his essential elements for a successful alternative as follows:

- *Choice* – No mandates. Using a system similar to Medicare, he advocates guaranteed insurance with community rating (the same premiums regardless of pre-existing medical conditions). But if you don't sign up when you're first eligible, you pay a penalty that may reflect your health status.
- *Fairness* – Annual tax credit of $2500 for every adult and $1500 for every child. The credit is available for anyone purchasing health insurance wherever it is purchased. No income means testing. This makes enrollment easy by removing all of the income data verification necessary in ObamaCare.
- *Jobs* – No disincentives for hiring means job expansion is unimpeded. No need to reduce workers to part-time hours or keep companies smaller. Also, with tax credits the incentive for purchasing higher cost insurance is removed. This lowers

employer costs for most companies and raises revenue from those who choose to purchase expensive insurance.

How *The Patient CARE Act* Is Better Than Obamacare

	Obamacare	Patient CARE Act
Reduces Rising Health Insurance Premiums	NO	YES
Allows Medicaid Beneficiaries Option to Purchase Private Coverage	NO	YES
Tax Credits are Received by the Patient (Not the Insurer)	NO	YES
Protects Rights of Conscience	NO	YES
New Taxes on Medical Devices, Prescription Drugs	YES	NO
Creates a New Government Website	YES	NO
Implements Federally-Run Health Exchanges in States	YES	NO
Federally-Defined Health Benefits	YES	NO
Creates a Board of Unelected Officials to Regulate Payments (IPAB)	YES	NO
Funds Federal Comparative Effectiveness Research	YES	NO
Restricts Health Savings Accounts and Flexible Savings Accounts	YES	NO
Expands a Broken Medicaid System	YES	NO
Provides for Special Treatment of Union Health Plans	YES	NO
Expands Health Tax Credits to Families Making More than $90,000	YES	NO
Covers Americans with Pre-Existing Conditions	YES	YES
Eliminates Lifetime Limits on Benefits	YES	YES
Provides Coverage for Dependents (Up to Age 26)	YES	YES

Figure 1– Comparison of The Patient CARE Act to ObamaCare. *Coburn.Senate.Gov*

- *Universality* – Everyone is eligible to purchase insurance with the tax credits. For those who don't, the money saved by the government should be sent to community-based healthcare institutions to provide care for the uninsured. This should ensure universal access to health care. He would also allow anyone who chooses to enroll in Medicaid; and everyone in Medicaid to leave the program to take advantage of the tax credit and purchase private insurance.

- **Portability** – Insurance should follow employees. When they change jobs the insurance goes with them, much like a 401K retirement plan does today. This solves the pre-existing medical conditions problem.
- **Patient Power** – Health Savings Accounts (HSAs) should be encouraged by making them completely flexible – and allowed to partner with third-party insurance in innovative ways. These accounts make savings possible up to 30 percent according to a RAND Corporation study. They empower and encourage patients to make better health care choices.
- **Real Insurance** – ObamaCare is mostly increasing the number of insured Americans by expanding Medicaid and enrolling people in low-cost plans available on the exchanges that have "narrow networks" that exclude the best doctors and hospitals (who won't accept the lower rates). Some have called these plans "Medicaid Plus".

Both of these situations may actually *decrease access* to healthcare for those previously uninsured. A solution to this problem is plans like the current Medicare Advantage plans that accept all comers but premiums are *not* community rated. As a result, insurance plans compete to enroll these patients instead of trying to avoid the sick. ObamaCare, however, is cutting funding for these plans despite their popularity with patients and insurance companies.

The 2017 Project

There are many good minds working on alternatives to ObamaCare. Among these are the founders of The 2017 Project, including Executive Director Jeffrey H. Anderson, writer for *The Weekly Standard,* and William Kristol, Editor of the same publication. Also instrumental in the development of their plan is James Capretta, Senior Fellow with The

Ethics and Public Policy Center. Their proposal, *A Winning Alternative to ObamaCare,* puts forth reasonable and workable solutions to the problems of ObamaCare that all Americans can and should endorse.

They identify the three core concerns of our healthcare system: the large number of **people without insurance**, the plight of the **uninsured with pre-existing expensive medical conditions**, and the **high cost of care**. They propose solutions to all three concerns in a "three legged" approach that takes advantage of the best of the previous conservative approaches put forth to date.

The *First Leg* is ending the unfairness of the tax code by offering *tax credits to the uninsured and the individually insured*. This approach is similar to Goodman's by providing universal tax credits that are *not means tested* – no income qualification or verification needed. They do have a sliding scale of credit by age ranging from a beginning tax credit of $1200 for those under age 35, to $2100 for those between ages 35 and 50, to $3000 for those ages 50 or over. In addition they give $900 per child.

These credits are only available on the individual market, unlike Goodman whose credits are available in any market. Those who purchase more expensive insurance would have to supplement their premiums. Those who purchase less expensive coverage could put the extra into an HSA account.

The Government Accountability Office (GAO) reports that these tax credits would be sufficient to purchase insurance through the individual market with no more than a $15/month supplementation in all but five states; the liberal havens of Maine, Massachusetts, New Jersey, New York, or Rhode Island. Smokers would pay more in some other states. However, with new regulations to permit the purchase of insurance across state lines, these differences would be moot.

The *Second Leg* addresses the problem of pre-existing conditions. It creates a *"buy in" period of the uninsured*; a grace period when they can purchase insurance and not be denied coverage due to pre-existing conditions. However, to prevent the gaming of the system, those who fail to enroll during this grace period will pay higher premiums if they enroll later. They would also have a two-month grace period if they change jobs and lose their employer-provided insurance. They would also propose state-run "high risk pools" to cover those with expensive medical conditions with federally provided subsidies.

The **Third Leg** would seek to lower the high cost of healthcare by *expanding the use of HSA accounts*. They would provide a one-time $1000 tax credit ($2000 per couple and $4000 for a family of four) for anyone establishing an HSA account. They would also cap the tax exclusion for employer-sponsored plans at the 75th percentile with a 3% annual escalation. This would incentivize employers to reduce costs while also providing revenue to pay for the plan from those who insist on purchasing these high cost plans.

Political Reality

Conservative writer and talk-show host William F. Buckley, Jr. wanted to elect conservative candidates. But he had a practical view when it came to choosing candidates to nominate. He said,

"The wisest choice would be the one who would win. No sense running Mona Lisa in a beauty contest. I'd be for the most right, viable candidate who could win. If you could convince me that Barry Goldwater could win, I'd vote for him."
— William F. Buckley Jr., 1967

When it comes to choosing an alternative to ObamaCare, Buckley's advice is good to remember. We must choose the most right, viable alternative that can gain bipartisan support.

Any of the alternatives we have discussed thus far would be a vast improvement over ObamaCare. But some would be attacked by the left for touching "third-rail" issues like reforming Medicare or malpractice reform. Others tamper with the tax deductions for employer-provided insurance. It is better to choose an alternative that does the most good possible – without creating such animosity on the left that it cannot pass in the Congress. Purists may find this approach squeamish but there is no use in a proposal that has no chance of ever becoming law.

The 2017 Project "three legged" approach keeps this principle in mind. It achieves three important elements in a winning political alternative.

First, a winning alternative must be something that can be sold to the American people on the political stump. In other words, it must be easy to describe in short "sound-bites" people can understand and the media can reproduce.

Second, it cannot afford to invite a political backlash by proposing ideas that are lightning rods for criticism. They believe it should not veer into important but nevertheless tangential issues like Medicare reform, and it shouldn't threaten the existence of the tax break for those with employer-provided health insurance. They do acknowledge, however, that it can – and should – prevent that tax break from being an open-ended public subsidy for ever-more-expensive plans.

Third, and most importantly, it must meaningfully address Americans' trio of core goals for real health-care reform: lowering costs, dealing with pre-existing conditions, and significantly increasing the number of people who are insured versus the pre-ObamaCare status quo.

Failing to offer solutions to each of these core concerns is the easiest way for a conservative alternative to become a target for criticism.

The Political Viability Debate

Democrats like to criticize Republicans for failure to put forward a unified alternative to ObamaCare. President Obama is the leader of this criticism:

"The only alternative that ObamaCare's critics have is, well, 'Let's just go back to the status quo, because they sure haven't presented an alternative.'"

President Barack Obama, press conference, December 2013

As we have seen already in this chapter, there are plenty of Republican alternatives that have been put forward. But, to be sure, there is still no consensus on the best approach.

Reasons for this include the lack of a singular party leader, as every party lacks when they do not occupy the White House. Republican candidates for the presidency hold back their views until they declare their candidacy and then try to separate themselves from the field by their unique proposals.

There is also a widely held view that coming forward with one particular alternative proposal presents a target for liberal criticism. Those who hold this view preferred to keep back the details until after the mid-term elections – thereby denying Democrats an election campaign issue. When the 2016 presidential campaign heats up, look for Republican candidates to come forward with their proposals.

Peter Ferrara

There is no shortage of debate about conservative alternatives to ObamaCare in the healthcare blogosphere. Prominent among these writers is Peter Ferrara, economist writer for *Forbes*. Ferrara has written widely on ObamaCare and has analyzed the alternatives already presented in this chapter.

Ferrara commends the 2017 Project proposal on many points. He agrees that any viable proposal to replace ObamaCare must significantly increase the number of insured Americans. He believes, as they do, that ObamaCare fails to create a true marketplace for healthcare insurance due to its top-down, bureaucratic solution with all of the critical decisions made in Washington. What is needed is a decentralized approach with consumers driving the system by the decisions they make about insurance coverage and the use of medical services.

He also believes, as do Capretta and others, that the open-ended tax subsidization of employer-paid health insurance is one of the main distortions of the existing system. This system encourages excessively costly employer plans and discriminates against households that do not have access to employer coverage and thus must rely on the individual market for insurance. There is no need for taxpayers to subsidize the cost of expensive health insurance policies.

However, he parts opinion with these writers when it comes to the best way to revise the employer-provided insurance system. Ferrara sides with the Goodman proposal in preferring tax credits for everyone – regardless of income level or employment status. He rejects the 2017 Project proposal that gives tax credits *only* to those purchasing insurance on the individual market. He believes that allowing workers with employer insurance to choose their own insurance they prefer with the tax credit empowers workers with an important check and balance of their employer choosing insurance that may be better for the employer but not for the workers.

James Capretta

Capretta argues that their approach is more politically viable. He believes it is bad politics to tamper with the currently existing employer-provided insurance system. In 2008, Senator John McCain proposed the full conversion to tax credits in the presidential campaign as was attacked relentlessly by the Obama-Biden campaign for unraveling employer-based insurance. These unfounded criticisms were nevertheless effective and contributed to Democratic momentum in this closely contested election.

Capretta responds:

"The attacks were hard to deflect in 2008, and would be again in 2014 or 2016, because the full switch to universal tax credits would lessen employer control over their workplace insurance plans. Many employers fear that, with a Ferrara-like universal credit, their younger, healthier workers will choose to buy low-cost plans on the individual market and leave employers with just the older and less healthy employees in their plans. Under this scenario, premiums for employer plans would rise rapidly. Anticipating this, many, if not most, large employers would oppose such an alternative, thereby diminishing the prospects for repeal."

Capretta, and the 2017 Project, are influenced by the same principles expressed above by William F. Buckley, Jr. They want an alternative that can win bipartisan support. The McCain experience has already shown the failure of a plan that tampers with the best of our current system – the employer-provided health insurance. That system provides insurance for 160 million Americans and most were quite happy with their plans (before ObamaCare cancelled them). The 2017 Project seeks to improve what is failing while holding on to what is working.

Ferrara also warns of a political risk associated with putting an upper limit on the tax break for employer coverage. The Patient CARE Act of Senators Coburn, Burr, and Hatch initially had an upper limit of 65% of an expensive employer-sponsored plan. This effectively creates a 35% tax for many middle to upper-income workers. Although this is less than the 40% "Cadillac tax" on ObamaCare plans after 2018, it is still a substantial increase over the current situation.

After initial introduction, however, the Senators discovered such a limit would actually produce large excess revenues and therefore they raised the cap so that it affects only the most expensive employer-sponsored plans.

The upper limit thresholds in the 2017 Project plan are about $8,000 for individuals and $20,000 for families. With these caps, only the most expensive plans would exceed these thresholds. Workers would still get generous subsidization of their health insurance but not for the premiums above the tax preference limits. In comparison, this is a less punitive cap than the ObamaCare "Cadillac tax".

The thoughtfulness of the 2017 Project proposal, and its reality-based understanding of what wins in today's political and media climate, impress me. As an orthopedic surgeon, I wish any new proposal would address the issue of malpractice reform. It is estimated that defensive medicine costs us over $60 billion annually. Yet I understand the "lightning rod" nature of that issue which is probably best left to individual states to address. It is better we fix the system as a whole first, then address more contentious issues in the future.

Currently, the Senate plan of Coburn-Burr-Hatch has the most support in Congress. But the improvements recommended by Goodman and the 2017 Project are substantial and should be seriously considered. The key features of a credible alternative have emerged as follows:

- **A commitment to market-driven health care**

    ObamaCare creates a government-imposed cost-control system – at the expense of a well-functioning marketplace. You can't have both. With federal control over the system, the free market cannot function and produce higher quality and lower costs. By the creation of a true marketplace, consumers will control the allocation of medical resources and create competition that drives down prices and raises quality.

- **Retention of employer-based coverage**

    By retaining the popular employer-based system of health insurance coverage you will largely satisfy the 160 million Americans currently receiving their insurance this way. This makes the plan politically viable. Both the Coburn-Burr-Hatch plan and The 2017 Project do this. Both cap the upper limit of tax exclusion on expensive plans.

- **Tax Credits for those without access to employer coverage**

    This levels the playing field for those without access to employer coverage. This approach is preferable to proposals that allow taxpayers to deduct the cost of insurance. A deduction's value is higher for higher-income taxpayers because they would pay higher tax rates on income excluded from taxes. A credit provides the same value to *all* taxpayers, regardless of income. The Coburn-Hatch-Burr plan is a *means-tested* tax credit while the 2017 Project and Goodman Proposal offers tax credits to everyone.

- **Continuous coverage protection**

    This retains the popular portion of ObamaCare that solves the problem of pre-existing medical conditions. However, unlike ObamaCare, these plans prevent people from "gaming the system" by signing up for coverage after they get sick. By providing a "grace period" of two months for anyone losing their coverage, patients can be sure they will find coverage even if they change jobs and lose their insurance. However, an even better solution is making insurance plans portable like 401K plans.

- **Better health care for the poor**

ObamaCare expands the rolls of Medicaid but does nothing to improve the access and quality of healthcare for those with that type of insurance. In fact, the Medicaid system will be even worse as it grows because of increased number of patients seeing a declining number of doctors. By providing tax credits to all those without employer-based insurance, many of those with Medicaid will find better, affordable care on the insurance exchanges. When the poor are able to enroll in the same insurance plans as higher-income workers they will achieve better access to doctors – and better healthcare outcomes.

Table One - Republican Alternatives to ObamaCare
Robert S. Roberts, M.D. – 10/16/14

Policy	Price	Roe	Coburn	Goodman	2017
• Insurance sold across state lines	Y	Y	Y	Y	Y
• Small business pools	Y	Y	Y	?	?
• Tax deductions	Y	Y	N	N	N
• Tax credits/ Refundable tax credits	Y	N	Y*	Y**	Y**
• *Malpractice caps on non-economic damages*	N	Y	N	N	Y
• *"Best practice guidelines"*	Y	N	N	N	N
• *Raise HSA limits*	N	Y	Y	Y	Y
• High risk pools for pre-existing conditions	Y	Y	Y	Y	Y

• Portable insurance policies	Y	Y	Y	Y	Y
• Prohibit federal funding of abortion	Y	Y	Y	?	?
• Repeal ObamaCare	Y	Y	Y	Y	Y
• Caps on Tax Exclusion	N	N	Y	Y	Y

* - means tested

** - *not* means tested

Price (GA) – Empowering Patients First Act (EPFA) – HR 2300

Roe (TN) – American Health Care Reform Act (AHCRA) – HR 3121

Coburn (OK) – Patient CARE Act – Senate proposal

Table Two - Key Differences

Policy	Price	Roe	Coburn	Goodman	2017
• Tax deductions	Y	Y	N	N	N
• *Tax credits/ Refundable tax credits*	Y	N	Y*	Y**	Y**
• *Malpractice caps on non-economic damages*	N	Y	N	N	Y
• *Raise HSA limits*	N	Y	Y	Y	Y
• *Caps on Tax Exclusion*	N	N	Y	Y	Y

* - means tested

** - *not* means tested

Price (GA) – Empowering Patients First Act (EPFA) – HR 2300

Roe (TN) – American Health Care Reform Act (AHCRA) – HR 3121

Coburn (OK) – Patient CARE Act – Senate proposal

Table One shows a comparison of these plans side-by-side. Table Two helps identify the key differences between the plans. In truth, the differences appear insignificant in these tables. But the political and economic consequences could be dramatic.

The Roy Proposal

Another alternative proposal comes from Avik Roy, long-time healthcare blogger and Senior Fellow at The Manhattan Institute. On 8/13/14 he published his health reform proposal entitled "*Transcending ObamaCare: A Patient-Centered Plan for Near-Universal Coverage and Permanent Fiscal Solvency.*" Roy has been a critic of ObamaCare for a long time and has been particularly vocal about the adverse impact of expanding care under Medicaid. He refers to Medicaid as "*the worst health insurance program in the developed world.*"

Roy's proposal draws heavily upon successful health insurance programs in other parts of the world, especially Switzerland and Singapore. These two countries spend far less on healthcare than the United States yet achieve near universal care.

Figure 2 shows the United States spends an average of $4,160 per capita while Switzerland spends $1,879 per capita and Singapore only $851 per capita. While spending levels alone do not necessarily reflect quality of care delivered, these figures represent large differences between three highly developed nations. The U.S. spends more than twice as much as Switzerland and nearly five times as much as Singapore.

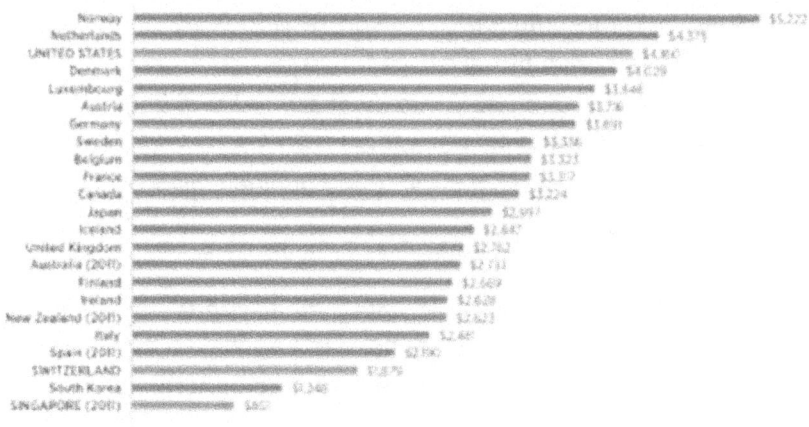

2012 Public Health Expenditure per Capita
(US$ purchasing power parity-adjusted)

Figure 2– Public Health Expenditures per Capita by country for 2012.

The Roy Proposal was developed by The Manhattan Institute for Policy Research in partnership with Stephen Parente, health economist at the University of Minnesota. The proposal established five non-negotiable goals as follows:

1. *Reduce the deficit without raising taxes*
2. *Expand coverage meaningfully above ACA levels*
3. *Repeal the Individual Mandate*
4. *Reduce the cost of private health insurance*
5. *Improve health outcomes for the poor*

Roy seeks to amend, rather than replace, ObamaCare by borrowing from these other market-driven healthcare systems. Switzerland offers premium subsidies to approximately one fifth of the population. By his calculations, the U.S. actually gives subsidies to four-fifths. He calls this the difference between a safety net and an entitlement leviathan.

The Roy Proposal is a four-step plan to take the entire collection of government health care programs and reform them into something consumer-driven and fiscally sustainable:

1. *Deregulate ObamaCare's insurance exchanges and repeal the Individual Mandate, while preserving guaranteed issue for individuals with pre-existing conditions*
2. *Migrate future retirees onto the reformed exchanges*
3. *Repeal ObamaCare's Employer Mandate*
4. *Migrate Medicaid acute-care and dual-eligible enrollees onto the exchanges*

He believes this would transform ObamaCare into a system much like Switzerland's. Rises in premium subsidies could be held to a sustainable growth rate to ensure their long-term stability. The goal is to give Americans the opportunity to purchase insurance for themselves, gain control of their own healthcare dollars, and enjoy a wide range of low-cost, high-quality coverage options.

Cost Comparisons with ObamaCare

How do these alternatives compare with the cost of ObamaCare? ObamaCare is expected to cost over $2 Trillion dollars from 2015 to 2024 according to the Congressional Budget Office (CBO). Over 90 percent of this amount, $1.863 Trillion would come in the form of direct spending or new outlays. The **2017 Project** proposal is estimated to cost $977 Billion – and most of that "cost" would come in the form of a tax cut. In direct spending terms, the cost is only $399 Billion over the decade – a savings of $1.464 Trillion compared to ObamaCare!

The **Coburn–Burr–Hatch** bill in the Senate was scored by the Center for Health and Economy, run by former CBO director Douglas Holtz-Eakin. They estimate a savings of $1.473 Trillion over the next ten years. They see the greatest deficit reduction in the caps on tax exclusion of employer-sponsored insurance plans. Some have labeled this a "big tax hike" and this portion of their plan is certainly that. But the plan still delivers $416 Billion in deficit reduction even if this portion of the plan is eliminated. In reality, there is no reason for the federal government (actually the taxpayers) to fund more and more expensive insurance policies as a way of employers increasing benefits without paying taxes.

The **Roy** proposal was scored by Stephan Parente, economist at The University of Minnesota. He calculates the plan, over a *thirty-year* period, reduces federal spending by $10.5 Trillion and federal revenues by $2.5 Trillion, for a net deficit reduction of $8 Trillion. They project that it will expand coverage by more than 12 million individuals over its first decade, despite the fact that it repeals the Individual Mandate. It reduces the cost of private-sector insurance policies by 17 percent for single policies and 4 percent for family policies.

Cost/Savings Comparison of Alternative Plans
Robert S. Roberts, M.D. – 10/16/14

Plan	Cost/2015-2024 (Trillions)	Savings/2015-2024 (Trillions)
ObamaCare	$1.863	-
2017 Project	$0.399	$1.464
Coburn	$0.390	$1.473
Roy	$1.834 *	$0.029 *#

* - 2016-2025 estimate
# - $8.0 Trillion savings for 2016 - 2045

Figure 3 – Cost and Savings Comparison of Alternative Plans.

They are most excited, however, about the impact of this plan on Medicaid. They believe there will be a dramatic increase in provider access and health outcomes, based on Parente-developed indices that measure these things. This improvement in Medicaid is based on the plan to give Medicaid patients the ability to purchase private health insurance with higher provider fees that will improve access to providers (doctors and hospitals) similar to those with private health insurance today.

New Scoring of 2017 Project

The scoring of the 2017 Project in the figures above comes from their internal estimates. Recently they received an independent scoring from the non-partisan Center for Health and Economy (H & E) founded by former Congressional Budget Office director Douglas Holtz-Eakin. The key findings of the H & E scoring are as follows:

- The 2017 Project's Alternative would save **$1.13 Trillion** in federal spending versus ObamaCare from 2014 through 2023.
- **Six million more Americans would have private health insurance** under the Alternative than under ObamaCare.
- Under the Alternative, premiums would decrease in the individual market "in all plan categories for both single and family coverage," with reductions ranging form 4 to 25 percent.
- Provider access – "access to desired physicians and facilities" – in the individual market would increase by 19 percent in the first year of the Alternative and by 57 percent as of 2023.
- Provider access in the employer-based market would increase by 4 percent.
- Medical productivity – the "efficient use of resources" – would increase by 10 percent in 2016 and would remain at about that level.
- **Twelve million fewer people would be on Medicaid**, and 6 million people who would have been put on Medicaid under ObamaCare would buy private insurance under the Alternative.
- ObamaCare would cover 249 million people, while the Alternative – without imposing an individual or employer mandate – would cover 243 million, thereby leaving 38 million uninsured under ObamaCare (13 percent of the population) versus 44 million under the Alternative (15 percent of the population) – with all of ObamaCare's additional coverage coming from increasing the Medicaid rolls.
- **ObamaCare would cover 6 million more people (all on Medicaid)** than the Alternative but would cost $1.13 Trillion more than the Alternative, which works out to $188,000 per additional covered person.
- The Alternative wouldn't needlessly disrupt the employer-based market – 149 million people would have employer-based insurance in 2015 (the year before the Alternative

would take effect), and the same number would have it in 2023 (the last year of the scoring).

- The Alternative would promote the purchase of genuine insurance while increasing the use of HSA accounts, thereby encouraging people to shop for value: "*The structure of the Alternative's premium credits encourage many catastrophic coverage enrollment, as households can purchase catastrophic plans for less than the value of the tax credits,*" with their savings going into HSAs.

- **In summary, the 2017 Project Alternative would:**
    o *Cut federal spending by over a trillion dollars*
    o *Increase the number of Americans with private insurance*
    o *Reduce premiums*
    o *Improve medical productivity*
    o *Enhance access to doctors and hospitals in both the individual and employer markets*

Burr-Hatch-Upton (Patient CARE II)

Shortly before this book went to print, a new proposal was introduced in the now Republican-controlled Congress. Senators Richard Burr and Orrin Hatch joined with Representative Fred Upton to propose a revised Patient CARE plan. (Senator Tom Coburn retired at the end of 2014.) This newly revised plan has been referred to as Burr-Hatch-Upton or Patient CARE II.

The new plan has the same tax credits as the old plan which are *means-tested.* They provide a sliding scale of tax-credits by income level and age beginning with individuals ages 18 – 34 year-olds earning less than 200% of the FPL. The top of the scale is families ages 50 – 64 years-old earning up to 300% of FPL.

The old plan was criticized for its high tax increase on employer-provided insurance since it capped the tax exclusion at 65% of an average plan's cost. The new plan is designed to be tax-neutral. It does this by raising the ceiling on the tax exclusion of employer-provided plan to $12,000 for individuals and $30,000 for families. This threshold will grow at Consumer Price Index plus 1 percent annually. By comparison, ObamaCare's "Cadillac tax" has a ceiling of $10,200 for individuals and $27,500 for families.

As a result of these changes the value of the tax credits under Burr-Hatch-Upton are 26% higher than under Coburn-Burr-Hatch. For example, under the old plan, a 40-year-old making less than 200 percent of FPL would receive a tax credit worth $2,530. Under the new plan, the tax credit would be worth $3,190.

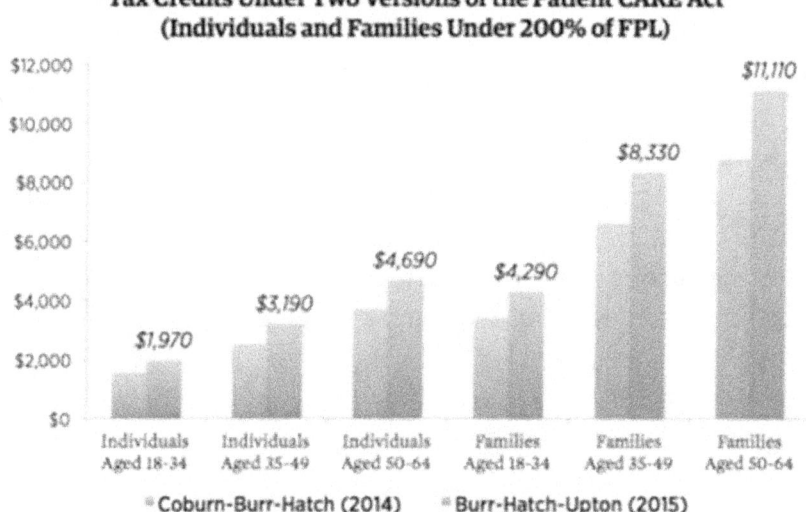

**Tax Credits Under Two Versions of the Patient CARE Act
(Individuals and Families Under 200% of FPL)**

Increased Coverage of the Uninsured

There's more good news. With these higher tax credits, this plan will surely cover more of the uninsured. Although the new plan has not been scored as of this writing, the old plan was scored by Parente et al. of the Center for Health and Economy and found to cover *3 million more people than ObamaCare*. The new plan will definitely exceed these impressive numbers.

Medicaid and Medicare Reform

Patient CARE II also addresses entitlement reform. It repeals ObamaCare's Medicaid expansion, allowing eligible individuals to instead use tax credits to purchase private insurance. Also, the plan adapts a 2013 proposal form Upton and Hatch to convert the Medicaid program into a "per-capita cap" – similar to block grants first proposed by President Bill Clinton.

Medical Malpractice Reform

Patient CARE II seeks to "combat junk lawsuits and reduce the practice of defensive medicine." It does this by proposing caps on non-economic damages and limits attorney's fees in medical liability cases. These measures have been successful in some states, such as Texas, in reducing medical malpractice claims.

Price Transparency

In order to encourage consumer-driven health care, Patient CARE II requires that hospitals accepting Medicare disclose the "average amount paid by uninsured and insured patients for the most common inpatient and outpatient procedures, among other things.

Interstate Insurance Purchasing

To increase competitive pricing of insurance policies, this plan "removes federal barriers that currently make it harder for Americans to buy coverage across state lines." This reform has been estimated to reduce health insurance costs by 9 percent.

Comparison of Plans

All of these plans would lower costs, increase the number of Americans with private insurance, lower premiums, improve access to providers, and replace government control of healthcare with private market-based reforms. The question becomes which one is best – and which one can win approval?

As I mentioned above, we need an alternative that can weather the storms of the political world to win bipartisan support. That must be the measuring stick for determining which plan conservatives should support.

Democrats might favor the reforms suggested by Avik Roy because they do not require the repeal of ObamaCare. His plan is largely based on reforms of the state-based insurance exchanges to raise the quality of their plans and provide tax credits to more people so they can purchase them. He would transition many people currently on Medicaid to these plans in this way. The system would resemble that found in Switzerland, to a large extent.

But others, including myself, are skeptical of retaining ObamaCare's core, which still maintains government control. Capretta has written his concern that the ObamaCare exchanges were built to assert increasing federal regulatory control over the nation's health system; a control not easily relinquished. He says,

"Even if a deregulation effort partially succeeds in the short run, over the long run, federal regulatory agencies gain power by cleverly creating vested interests in the protection and expansion of that power. It is a very risky bet to place the future of American health care at the mercy of a new and improved system of ObamaCare exchanges."

The Coburn-Burr-Hatch (Patient CARE) plan has been criticized for its ceiling on employer-provided tax exclusion at 65% of the average plan premium. This was criticized as a 35% tax on *average* plan premiums. But the new Burr-Hatch-Upton plan reduces this impact to even less than ObamaCare. This reduces the revenues from the plans, which were substantial, and applies the exclusion only to the most expensive plans available. With this significant change, their proposal is fiscally sound and politically viable.

The Patient CARE II plan does limit tax credits to those who earn 300% of the Federal Poverty Level (FPL) or less. The ObamaCare subsidies go up to 400% of FPL. Both necessitate income verification, which has greatly complicated the process of enrollment and contributed to the crash of the government web site. The Goodman and 2017 Project plans eliminate this problem by giving everyone a tax credit; without qualification in the Goodman plan and if an employer-based plan is unavailable in the 2017 Project plan. This is simpler than the Patient CARE plan.

Lastly, the 2017 Project plan could be criticized for insuring 6 million fewer Americans than ObamaCare (all of them on Medicaid), although it increases the number on private insurance by the same number of 6 million. Capretta addresses this criticism by conceding the issue, but offering a simple solution by including a "default enrollment" provision similar to what is included in the Coburn-Burr-Hatch plan.

Although the plan calls for a tax credit for every household without access to an employer plan, the H & E scoring assumes that millions of these households will decline to use the credit to buy any kind of health insurance product. A "default enrollment" provision would automatically enroll those who failed to choose a product – at no cost to the enrollees. (They would be enrolled in plans where the tax credits exactly equaled the premium costs.) This would eliminate the disparity in the number of insured compared to ObamaCare.

The 2017 Project also caps the tax-exclusion for employer-based plans but does so at 75% of the cost of expensive plans. This is a higher cap than Coburn-Burr-Hatch, which means it raises slightly less revenue but is even more politically correct. It is not as high as the new Burr-Hatch-Upton plan.

James Capretta summarizes the situation:

"It's time – long past time – for ACA opponents to begin coalescing around something that is realistic, politically and substantively. The H & E estimates make it clear that a synthesis of Coburn-Burr-Hatch and the 2017 Project would do the trick."

Means-tested v. Uniform Tax Credits

The most contentious issue being debated among conservative reformers is between *means-tested tax credits* and *uniform tax credits.* Means-tested tax credits are only available to those earning less than a determined income ceiling. Uniform tax credits are available to everyone, regardless of income.

Both Burr-Hatch-Upton and the Roy Plan prefer *means-testing.* Roy argues this takes into account the fact that we already massively subsidize health coverage for upper-income folks, through the employer tax exclusion and Medicare. These plans offer the attractive benefit of increasing coverage of the uninsured – beyond ObamaCare.

Those plans taking a *uniform* tax credits approach include The 2017 Project and the Goodman Proposal. They argue a means-tested approach represents a tax on earning more money and discourages more work. Furthermore, this represents another income redistribution plan like so much of the Obama administration policies. Lastly, this simplifies the enrollment online because there is no need for income verification.

Comparing the Replace Plans vs. ACA

	Roy / Manhattan Institute	Burr-Hatch-Upton	Anderson / 2017 Project
Compatible with repeal & replace	Yes	Yes	Yes
Requires repeal of Obamacare	No	Yes	Yes
Medicare reform	Yes	Yes	No
Medicaid reform (of pre-ACA program)	Yes	Yes	No
Hospital monopoly reform	Yes	No	No
Tax credit comparison			
200% FPL, 41-year-old	$4,410	$3,190	$2,100
350% FPL, 41-year-old	$0	$0	$2,100
1000% FPL, 41-year-old	$0	$0	$2,100
Disruption of ACA-covered pop.	Minimized	Meaningful	Significant

Roy believes these plans provide too much help to upper-income individuals and not enough to the poor and middle class. Because they must distribute the tax credits over a larger population, the tax credits are smaller and therefore fewer people will be covered by insurance. The 2017 Project was scored by Stephen Parente and was estimated to cover 6 million fewer than ObamaCare. Roy believes these plans are not politically viable in an election year.

Means-Tested Tax Credits v.	**Uniform Tax Credits**
o Benefits poor and low-income	Benefits everyone
o Covers more people	Covers fewer people
o Discourages earning more money	Encourages earning more money
o Redistributes income	Avoids income redistribution
o More complex enrollment	Simpler enrollment
o Politically more attractive	Politically less attractive

This graphic outlines the pros and cons of *means-tested v. uniform* tax credits. Each has strengths and weaknesses. The last line, political attractiveness, may be the deciding issue, since no plan matters if it doesn't become law. Both will be an improvement over ObamaCare. Therefore, the one that can be passed by both houses of Congress and be signed by the president is the one that should be chosen.

An Election Test

In the November 2014 Mid-term elections, Republican Senate candidate Ed Gillespie nearly pulled off the biggest upset of the night in his race against popular incumbent Mark R. Warner. Gillespie got over a million votes running on a five-point plan for economic growth, and the first point was a specific proposal to replace ObamaCare.

Gillespie's plan was virtually identical to the plan proposed above by **The 2017 Project.** Perhaps the best illustration of the plan's attractiveness is a comparison of a typical family; first, with ObamaCare, and then, with the alternative plan: *"A household in Virginia of two 36 year-olds making $63,000 a year gets no subsidy under ObamaCare, but under my plan, they'd get a tax credit worth $4,200. And those with policies covering adult children up to their 26th birthday could keep them."*

Gillespie's unexpectedly strong showing in that election proves the American people are ready for an improved healthcare reform plan to replace ObamaCare. I believe Republicans should support an alternative similar to his plan.

Summary of Reforms

There is general agreement on many issues even among most Democrats.

Every alternative proposal advocates selling insurance across state lines to increase competition and lower premium costs. Every alternative encourages the formation of small business pools to give these employers the same pricing advantages as large employers. Every plan ensures that those Americans with pre-existing medical conditions will not be shut out of the healthcare insurance market. Every plan increases the number of Americans with health insurance.

What is new is the realization that tax credits are better than tax deductions because they provide the means to purchase insurance for Americans of all income levels. To provide the funds for such a program these recent proposals all place caps on the tax exclusion of employer-provided insurance. Even ObamaCare has a 40% surcharge tax on all insurance policies that exceed $10,200/year beginning in 2018.

The evolution of conservative alternatives has now produced proposals that improve upon the inadequacies and perverse incentives of ObamaCare, save Trillions of dollars over the next decade, and should garner broader support from conservatives, independents, and even liberals.

They provide *more coverage of more Americans, eliminate the problems of pre-existing medical conditions,* and *lower costs to both patients and the taxpayers.* What's more they do so with the *preservation of religious freedom and choice,* and without the takeover of one sixth of the economy by the federal government. What's not to like?

13

The Future of Medicare

"Thanks to the Affordable Care Act, we are taking important steps to improve the quality of care for Medicare beneficiaries, while improving Medicare's long-term solvency."
Marilyn Tavenner, Administrator
Centers for Medicare and Medicaid Services - 7/28/14

Readers of this book over the age of fifty-five begin this chapter with a heightened interest. If you're on Medicare now, or will be in the next ten years, you want to know what will happen to Medicare.

If you saw the press release quoted above from the administrator of the Centers for Medicare and Medicaid Services (CMS), you might think there's nothing to worry about. But if you've been paying attention to other claims from this administration about healthcare, you know you should be skeptical.

Healthcare economist John C. Goodman takes the CMS statement to task in a response printed in his *Forbes* healthcare blog. Goodman says:

"If a private pension fund made claims like this the Justice Department would probably have the guilty parties up on charges of fraud."

That's a long way from reassurance about the future of Medicare. So where does the truth lie between these two vastly different perceptions of the solvency of Medicare?

CMS Claims About Medicare

The CMS press release makes the following claims:

- Slower Medicare growth has added four more years to the life of the Medicare Trust Fund, relative to last year's report.
- The main reason is the Affordable Care Act (ObamaCare), including new payment methods the administration has been experimenting with and the establishment of Accountable Care Organizations (ACOs).

Goodman takes issue with both of these claims:

First, the Medicare Trust Fund, referred to in the first statement, is spoken of as if it was a real account with real money. But in reality it is just an empty box with a giant IOU placed there by the federal government. As Goodman puts it,

"Medicare, in other words, is run like a Bernie Madoff scheme. That's why it has a huge unfunded liability totaling trillions of dollars."

Goodman refers to the work of Devon Herrick, fellow writer for *Forbes,* who explains the projections of future spending:

"The Trustees Report is supposed to project future Medicare spending based on current law. But, that also means the official projection includes provisions meant to slow spending growth that the Trustees know are unlikely to occur. In years past, the Trustees tended to ignore these uncomfortable facts. Around 2010 the Office of the Actuary at CMS took the unprecedented step of producing an Alternative Scenario report explaining that the assumptions in the Trustees Report were unrealistic, and the projections were most assuredly wrong. That raised eyebrows in the policy world. This year, the alternatives scenarios (i.e. conditions that are more likely to occur) crept up from the appendix (at the back) and landed uncomfortably on page 2."

Figure 1 shows three projected lines for the growth of Medicare spending for the rest of the century. The lowest line, the one predicting the least spending, is the one CMS is using for their optimistic projections. The Trustees' Report, however, says the future spending is more likely to follow one of two higher rates over the next 50 or more years. They realistically state the following:

"Current law requires CMS to implement a reduction in Medicare payment rates for physician services of almost 21 percent in April 2015. However, it is a virtual certainty that lawmakers will override this reduction as they have every year beginning with 2003."

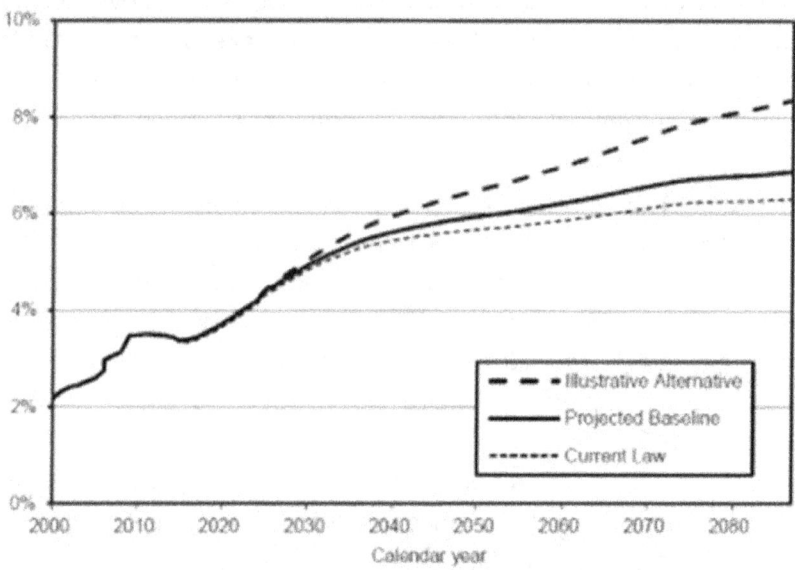

Figure 1 – Medicare Expenditures as a percentage of the Gross Domestic Product under Current Law, Projected Baseline, and Illustrative Alternative projections.

What is "Current Law?" It is ObamaCare. The provisions of the law call for a 21% reduction in provider fees to doctors and hospitals by April, 2015. However, the Trustees understand that these draconian reductions in fees to doctors will create havoc in the system as thousands of doctors refuse to see Medicare patients. To prevent this chaos, Congress will pass legislation, the so-called "doc fix" at the last minute, as they have every year since 2003.

Since 1997, the "Sustainable Growth Rate" (SGR) formula has been a part of Medicare. It is intended to control costs by automatically reducing reimbursement rates for doctors participating in the Medicare program. By reducing fees to doctors, the SGR holds down the growth of Medicare spending.

However, fees to doctors are so low already that in 2013, 28% of Medicare patients had difficulty finding a new doctor. If the SGR formula is allowed to take effect, that number will be even higher because doctors will have little incentive to take on new patients. Congress knows this, and hears frequently from senior constituents, so every year they pass legislation to temporarily prevent these cuts. This is called the "doc fix".

Thus, more realistic projections of Medicare spending take into account what is most likely to happen. By these more realistic projections, Medicare future spending follows the upper line in the graph, which is 50% higher than current law spending. Therefore, the press release of CMS administrator Tavenner is just putting "lipstick on a pig", to use a familiar phrase.

Second, the CMS report gives credit to ObamaCare for this supposed improvement in Medicare solvency. How has ObamaCare impacted the solvency of Medicare? The report gives credit to *"new payment methods the administration has been experimenting with and the establishment of ACOs."*

Once again, Goodman holds the CMS report accountable:

"We have spent tens of millions of dollars on demonstration programs and pilot projects investigating coordinated care, integrated care, managed care, pay-for-performance medicine, electronic medical records systems, etc. The result? Three separate Congressional Budget office reports have concluded that none of this is working, or at least not working very well.

The experience of the pilot ACO projects has been dismal. A total of 5.3 million Medicare beneficiaries are now in Medicare ACOs. Yet in their first year, only 29 percent of the physician-led ACOs and only

20 percent of the hospital-sponsored ACOs turned a "profit." And among those that did so, the results were fairly mediocre."

As discussed in Chapter Nine, the Medicare "Pioneer" ACO project originally featured 32 health systems hand-selected by HHS. In the first year, one third dropped out of the program. In year two, spending increased at six of the remaining 23 and only 11 received a bonus (meaning they met their benchmarks). Many dropped out because they figured out they could make more money outside the program. There is no evidence that ACOs have improved quality for seniors as the CMS press release purports.

The Medicare Trustees

We often talk about the "Medicare Trustees" without really knowing whom we're talking about. Who are these people who tell us not to worry about Medicare and spin the facts as we have just discussed?

The Medicare Trustees are composed of three cabinet positions appointed by the President, the Social Security Commissioner, and two public representatives, also appointed by the President. Current Medicare Trustees are:

- HHS Secretary Sylvia Matthews Burwell
- Treasury Secretary and Managing Trustee Jacob Lew
- Labor Secretary Thomas Perez
- Acting Social Security Commissioner Carolyn Colvin
- Public representative Charles Blahous III, Ph.D. – research fellow at Stanford's Hoover Institution
- Public representative Robert Reischauer, Ph.D. – economist and President Emeritus of the Urban Institute
- CMS Administrator Marilyn Tavenner is designated as Secretary of the Board

There can be no doubt that the three cabinet appointees and the Social Security Commissioner represent the Obama administration and have strong incentives to spin the facts to suit the White House's political agenda. While the public representatives are more independent, their minority vote on the Board is unlikely to influence the final report. The Office of the Actuary for Medicare is more independent and therefore has greater credibility.

Charles Blahous, however, has been an outspoken critic of ObamaCare and is referenced in the discussion of the costs of ObamaCare in Chapter Nine.

The Impact of the ACA on Medicare

We've discussed the problems of Medicare solvency, despite the claims of CMS and the Obama administration. But what impact has ObamaCare really had on the future of Medicare?

A Global Budget

For the first time in its history, Medicare is now on a global budget. ObamaCare imposes spending limits on Medicare. Until now, Medicare spent whatever was considered necessary to provide healthcare for seniors. Medical providers, doctors and hospitals and related medical services vendors, were paid according to legitimate bills submitted to Medicare. Spending increased or decreased according to the bills submitted.

But now ObamaCare has placed a ceiling on Medicare spending. For most of its history, per capita Medicare spending in real terms grew at about twice the rate of growth of real per capita GDP – just like the rest of the healthcare system. ObamaCare changes all that. The law requires Medicare to grow at a rate that is not much more than the growth of GDP – regardless of how spending grows in the rest of the healthcare system.

IPAB

ObamaCare creates a new government regulatory panel called the Independent Payment Advisory Board (IPAB), which is authorized to make cuts in Medicare spending. The board is composed of 15 individuals appointed by the President who will be given the power to make recommendations to cut Medicare spending beginning in January 2015. This body of unelected officials will make their recommendations based on the growth of Medicare spending. In each year that Medicare's per capita costs exceed a certain threshold, IPAB will be responsible for making proposals to reduce this projected cost growth to the specified threshold. The policies will then take effect automatically unless Congress specifically passes legislation blocking them and the president signs that legislation. This can only be done by a three-fifths "super-majority" vote.

The purpose of IPAB is to give political cover to the White House so that unpopular cuts in Medicare spending can be made without political repercussions. *These unelected officials will be unaccountable to the voters.*

ObamaCare stipulates that fewer than half of the 15 members of the IPAB can be involved in providing or managing the delivery of Medicare items and services, including healthcare providers. Furthermore, no member can serve as a practicing physician or be otherwise employed. Board members are appointed by the President but must be confirmed by the Senate.

As of this writing the President has not appointed anyone to IPAB. But the law stipulates that the HHS Secretary is a voting member of IPAB – and can act unilaterally if there are no other IPAB members appointed. Therefore, current HHS Secretary Sylvia Matthews Burwell has the power to make recommendations to cut Medicare spending *all by herself* – and it would take a "super-majority" of Congress to alter these recommendations.

Michael Cannon and Diane Cohen, healthcare analysts for The Cato Institute, have written extensively on IPAB. They are greatly concerned about this newly appointed panel that usurps the powers of Congress. They write:

"The Independent Payment Advisory Board is worse than unconstitutional—it is anti- constitutional. Congress's legislative powers do not include the power to alter the constitutional procedure

required for the passage of laws. Nor does it include the power to en-trench legislation by preventing it from being altered by future Congresses."

Cohen and Cannon say to call IPAB's recommendations "proposals" is misleading because they effectively have the force of law. The reasons for this are twofold:

- ObamaCare requires the HHS Secretary to implement them.
- ObamaCare severely restricts Congress's ability to reject them (they become law automatically unless Congress intervenes by a "super-majority").

It gets worse. Not only will IPAB's "proposals" effectively become law but ObamaCare has provisions built into it that will make it nearly impossible for future Congresses or Presidents to block these proposals. These provisions have the effect of eliminating any accountability to the people.

Cannon gives several reasons for this:

- **ObamaCare exempts the board's proposals from the rulemaking requirements** that Congress imposes on other executive branch agencies. The law does not require IPAB to hold hearings, take testimony, or receive evidence from the public.
- **ObamaCare authorizes IPAB to submit its proposals directly to Congress** as "legislative proposals." The President's constitutional authority is undermined by this provision because it removes his discretion on what legislation is submitted to Congress.
- **Once the legislative proposal is submitted to Congress, ObamaCare protects it** by codifying changes to the normal parliamentary rules that permit the Senate or the House of Representatives to modify the proposal. Then, if Congress

fails to pass an alternative proposal that achieves the same budgetary goal, the IPAB proposal becomes law automatically.

- **If Congress fails to repeal IPAB through the restrictive procedure laid out in the law, then after 2020, Congress loses the ability to even offer substitutes** for IPAB proposals. The HHS Secretary is then empowered to implement IPAB's proposals even if Congress does enact a substitute. To constrain IPAB at all, Congress must do so between January and August of 2017.
- **ObamaCare gives IPAB and the HHS Secretary the sole authority to judge their own actions** by prohibiting administrative or judicial review of the Secretary's implementation of an IPAB proposal.

How can this unconstitutional seizure of the authority of Congress and the President be stopped?

The law specifies precisely how IPAB can be repealed:

1. *Wait until the year 2017.*
2. *Introduce a specifically worded "Joint Resolution" in Congress, both the House and Senate, between January 1 and February 1, 2017.*
3. *Pass that resolution by a three-fifths "super-majority" vote in both the House and Senate by August 15, 2017.*
4. *The President must then sign the "Joint Resolution."*

This is more restrictive than any other federal legislation. Congress has the ability to repeal any federal statute at any time with just a simple majority vote in both chambers and the signature of the President.

But ObamaCare has created an independent advisory board that can effectively make laws that will affect all Americans. They can do so without the direct approval of Congress or the President. Furthermore, that board can only be repealed by a joint resolution of Congress introduced only within about 15 business days in the year 2017. Then it has only seven more months to decide once and for all and must do so with a three-fifths "super-majority' vote in both house of Congress.

Has Congress ever achieved such broad agreement on any comparable issue in modern history?

Cohen and Cannon point to the work of Friedrich Hayek, who in 1944 wrote the classic work on government intrusion into the private sector called *The Road to Serfdom.*

"The federal government's attempts to direct America's health care sector, up to and including IPAB, closely track the predictions Nobel laureate economist Friedrich Hayek made in his 1944 book **The Road to Serfdom**. *Hayek explained how government planning of the economy leads to frustration with democracy and support for authoritarian forms of government such as IPAB:*

"It may be the unanimously expressed will of the people that its parliament should prepare a comprehensive economic plan, yet neither the people nor its representatives need there-fore be able to agree on any particular plan. The inability of democratic assemblies to carry out what seems to be a clear mandate of the people will inevitably cause dissatisfaction with democratic institutions. Parliaments come to be regarded as ineffective "talking shops," unable or incompetent to carry out the tasks for which they have been chosen. The conviction grows that if efficient planning is to be done, the direction must be "taken out of politics" and placed in the hands of experts – permanent officials or independent autonomous bodies. . . .The delegation of particular technical tasks to separate bodies, while a regular feature, is yet only the first step in the process whereby a democracy which embarks on planning progressively relinquishes its powers."

Friedrich Hayek, 1944 – *The Road to Serfdom*

"Nearly eight decades before Peter Orszag (chief architect of IPAB) *argued that IPAB would "take some of the politics out" of government-run health care, Hayek presaged Orszag's argument almost verbatim."*

Challenges to IPAB

Currently there is a bill in the House of Representatives, HR 351 sponsored by Rep. Phil Roe (R – Tenn) and Rep. Allyson Schwartz (D – Penn), that seeks to overturn the legislation that permits the IPAB to function. According to a report by Kristin Leighty in *AAOS Now,* HR 351 now has 120 co-sponsors. There is also a bill in the Senate introduced by Senator John Cornyn (R – Texas) called the Protecting Seniors' Access to Medicare Act of 2013 which is co-sponsored by Sen. Orrin Hatch (R – Utah) and 30 other Republican senators. This bill parallels the HR 351 bill in the House. Both seek to repeal the IPAB. More than 25 medical societies support the HR 351 bill.

There is reason for some optimism of a successful repeal since a similar attempt last year, HR 5, initially drew many Democratic sponsors. However, when the bill was incorporated with medical malpractice reform, these sponsors withdrew their support. Although the bill passed in the House, it was not acted upon in the Senate.

On April 25, 2013, over 500 organizations representing patients, individuals with disabilities, the elderly, veterans, healthcare providers and employers sent a letter to Congress urging lawmakers to repeal the IPAB. The letter asserts that IPAB will have a harmful impact on Medicare beneficiaries' access to quality healthcare and also sets a dangerous precedent by essentially transferring legislative responsibilities to an unelected board that is not subject to judicial review.

"We are deeply concerned about the impact IPAB will have on patient access to quality healthcare," the letter states. *"The bulk of any recommended spending reductions will almost certainly come in the form of payment cuts to Medicare providers. This will affect patient access to care and innovative therapies."*

The letter cites an AMA survey showing that a significant number of physicians are already restricting the number of Medicare patients they see in their practices because of low reimbursement rates. Also mentioned in the letter is a CBO finding that IPAB will likely focus its recommendations on Medicare payment rates in order to achieve short-term scoreable savings.

IPAB is also being challenged in the courts. *Coons v. Lew* (formerly *Coons v. Geithner*) challenges the constitutionality of IPAB. This case is pending for review by the Ninth Circuit Court of Appeals in California. One of the plaintiffs, Eric Novack, a medical doctor, faces potential cuts in his reimbursement rates via IPAB decrees. His case is supported by the Goldwater Institute and challenges IPAB for violating the Constitution's separation of powers.

The brief submitted by the Goldwater Institute describes IPAB in these terms:

"IPAB represents the most comprehensive consolidation of executive, judicial, and legislative power in a single administrative entity in American constitutional history."

Quin Hillyer, columnist for *National Review Online*, points out the immense powers of IPAB to set policy for any matter *"related to the Medicare program"* with other provisions making clear that IPAB can treat within that purview any *"system-wide health-care costs, patient access to care, utilization, and quality of care. . . including from private payers."* He notes, *"It can do so without resorting to ordinary notice-and-comment rule-making and with very little opportunity for Congress to overturn its decisions or even amend them beyond a severely circumscribed scope. Worse, IPAB's actions are exempt from judicial review, leaving aggrieved parties with neither legislative, administrative, nor judicial recourse in reining in unwarranted power grabs."*

As of this writing, IPAB remains an integral part of ObamaCare and is unlikely to be removed by the Obama Administration. They consider it an important means of controlling escalating health care costs and have already rejected other cost-containment policies like expanding HSAs and giving consumers greater choices and providers greater incentives to offer competitive pricing and improved quality. However, the Obama Administration has not made any recommendations for IPAB members yet, which leaves HHS Secretary Burwell as the only active member of the board.

The Fate of Medicare Patients

How should seniors respond? The future of Medicare is bleak unless there are changes made. The path laid out by ObamaCare will bring declining payments to doctors and hospitals, which will mean seniors will have increasing difficulty finding someone to provide their healthcare. *Even the CMS actuaries predict fees to doctors and hospitals will fall below Medicaid rates by 2020.*

If that happens, everyone on Medicare will struggle to find a doctor, just as people on Medicaid do today. The quality of their healthcare will also begin to resemble Medicaid with longer waiting times to see a doctor – and increased likelihood to use emergency rooms for primary care.

Figure 2 depicts a comparison of Medicare, Medicaid, and private health insurance prices for physician services if ObamaCare remains unchanged in the future. The graph of Medicare payments is shown dipping below Medicaid and steadily declining thereafter:

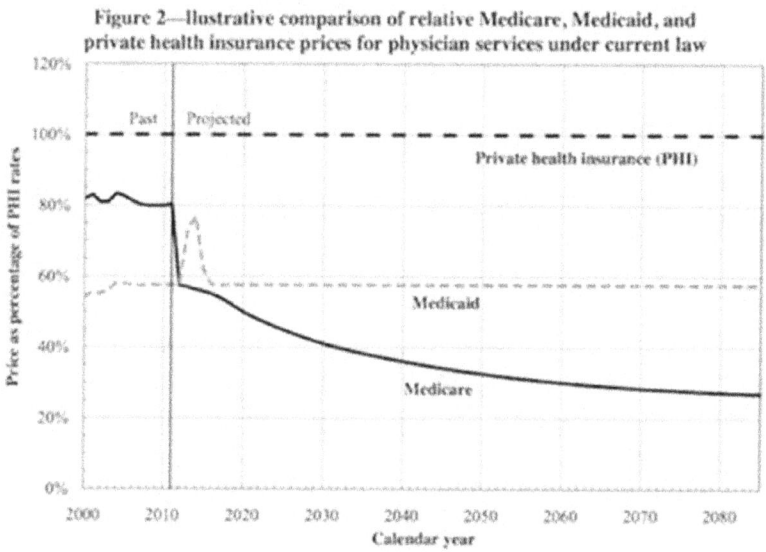

Figure 2—Illustrative comparison of relative Medicare, Medicaid, and private health insurance prices for physician services under current law

For wealthier seniors, the solution may be "concierge" medical practices. These primary care physicians offer greater access to the doctor and improved service after-hours in return for a monthly or yearly fee. Such practices are growing rapidly and will supply an increasing percentage of healthcare in the future. In several states, including California, Florida, Pennsylvania, and Virginia, surveys indicate that 90 percent of physicians are at least considering concierge medicine.

For lower-income seniors, the future will look much like Medicaid today. They will have to get used to second-class healthcare. Some may be able to put off this situation by maintaining employer-based health insurance as long as they are working. This may represent an increasingly important motivation for older workers to avoid retirement in the future – as long as possible.

Ultimately, the answer lies in repealing ObamaCare and passing new healthcare legislation that creates a level playing field for all Americans – regardless of their age, economic status, or current medical condition (Chapter Twelve).

The Gruber Tapes

"Lack of transparency is a huge political advantage."
MIT economist Jonathan Gruber
University of Pennsylvania conference - 10/ 17/13

In 1974 President Richard Nixon was forced to resign his presidency. After an audiotape was discovered of Oval Office conversations on July 23, 1972, six days after the infamous break-in at the Watergate complex, the world learned what the Nixon administration had been hiding.

In that tape, the so-called "smoking gun," Nixon agreed that administration officials should approach Richard Helms, Director of the CIA, and Vernon A. Walters, Deputy Director, and ask them to request L. Patrick Gray, Acting Director of the FBI, to halt the Bureau's investigation into the Watergate break-in on the grounds that it was a national security matter. The special prosecutor, Leon Jaworski, felt that Nixon, in so agreeing, had entered into a criminal conspiracy whose goal was the obstruction of justice.

The tape came from a system installed in the Oval Office by Nixon that was audio-activated and intended to record all conversations in that office. Only a select few individuals knew of the existence of the tapes. Little did Nixon expect that the installation of the system would eventually bring about his resignation.

Gruber Tapes Revealed

Recently a series of videotapes have been revealed that depict conversations by MIT economist Jonathan Gruber, one of the chief architects of ObamaCare. While these videotapes hardly represent an existential threat to the Obama administration and the presidency of Barack Obama, they definitely represent such a threat to his signature healthcare legislation.

The University of Pennsylvania Tape

The first of the tapes revealed was taken at The University of Pennsylvania on October 17, 2013. Speaking on a panel at a conference on healthcare economics, along with Penn health economist Mark Pauly, Gruber said:

"Mark (Pauly) made a couple of comments that I do want to take issue with, one about transparency in financing and the other is about moving from community rating to risk-rated subsidies. You can't do it politically. You just literally cannot do it, okay, transparent financing. . . and also transparent spending. In terms of risk-rated subsidies, if you had a law which said that healthy people are going to pay in – you made explicit that healthy people pay in and sick people get money, it would not have passed, okay. **Lack of transparency is a huge political advantage.** *And basically, call it the stupidity of the American voter or whatever, but basically that was really, really critical for the thing to pass. . . . Look, I wish Mark was right that we could make it all transparent, but I'd rather have this law than not."*

Gruber is admitting what the Obama administration will never admit – that they deceived the American people intentionally. The same president who often brags that his administration is *"the most transparent in history"* intentionally deceived voters so he could pass his healthcare legislation.

But wait, there's much more. Gruber then went on to explain why the bill was written in such a complicated way. He said:

"This bill was written in a tortured way to make sure CBO did not score the mandate as taxes. If CBO scored the mandate as taxes, the bill dies."

Now he is discussing the Individual Mandate, the portion of the law that requires everyone to purchase health insurance. Gruber claims credit for insisting a mandate to purchase health insurance was necessary in the law to prevent people from waiting until they get sick to purchase coverage. He was responsible for this mandate being written into the Massachusetts healthcare bill known as RomneyCare and he convinced President Obama it was needed in ObamaCare.

However, he also convinced President Obama not to call it a tax. This was in keeping with Obama's promises not to raise taxes on the middle class so he gladly promoted the Individual Mandate as a "penalty" rather than a tax. Gruber's confession simply confirms the reasoning behind the "tortured way" the bill was written.

History confirms the CBO did not score the mandate as a "tax" but the Supreme Court later ruled it was indeed a tax – and therefore was constitutional. But that ruling came two years after the law had already passed the Democratic-controlled Congress.

The Washington University Tape

Not long after the release of the tape from the University of Pennsylvania was revealed, a second tape was released. This was from another academic conference, also in October 2013 at Washington University in St. Louis. In this videotape Gruber discusses the so-called "Cadillac tax" portion of ObamaCare.

The "Cadillac tax", which begins in 2018, is a 40% tax added to the price of any healthcare insurance policy that exceeds $10,200 for individuals and $27,500 for families. Although the tax is levied on insurance companies, the impact will still be felt by the insured.

Gruber understands this well but doesn't credit the American people with the same understanding. He said:

"We just tax the insurance companies, they pass on higher prices that offsets the tax break we get, it ends up being the same thing. It's

a very clever, you know, basic exploitation of the lack of economic understanding of the American voter."

In another videotape on the same subject, Gruber explained his intent was to get rid of the tax-exclusion currently enjoyed by employer-provided health insurance. He estimated the amount of tax revenues forgone because of this exception to the usual rules for taxing compensation is at least $250 Billion per year.

Rather than simply take away the exclusion, which would be regarded as a huge tax increase on people, he concocted this alternative to deceive the voters. He explained that the only way to get rid of the tax preference for employer-sponsored insurance was *"by mislabeling it, calling it a tax on insurance plans rather than a tax on people, when we all know it's a tax on people who hold those insurance plans."*

The Impact of the "Cadillac Tax"

Tevi Troy, writing in *The Wall Street Journal,* released a study done with fellow economist Mark Wilson that shows Gruber is correct about the deceptive design of the "Cadillac tax." Rather than impacting only a few people with expensive plans, they say the tax is likely to hit many people who don't have high-end coverage.

Their study shows the cost increase will be passed on to employees or consumers in several ways. Large employers who are subject to the excise tax in 2018 will pay an average of more than $2700 per employee a year from 2018 to 2024. This cost will be passed on to consumers or to employees in higher prices and lower compensation. They explain:

"Employers, being rational actors, will not want to pay these taxes and will reduce their health-care benefits to limit their potential exposure to the tax. Doing this will cause employees to be hit by the excise tax in at least two other ways. If employers increase taxable wages to compensate for reducing the value of their plans, then employees will be paying more in taxes for the same compensation levels, and more after-tax out-of-pocket expenses for their heath care."

Their study calculates from 2018 to 2024 the excise tax could cost 12.1 million employees an average $1,050 in higher payroll and income taxes a year, if employers increase their taxable wages as they reduce the cost of health-care benefits. Alternatively, if employers only reduce the value of their insurance coverage without increasing wages and salaries, these employees could see up to a $6,150 reduction in their health-care benefits and little or no increase in pay.

Gruber understands all this and even acknowledges that the use of the term "Cadillac tax" is deceiving, too. He admits, *"Over time it's gonna apply to more and more health-insurance plans. . . The tax that starts out hitting only 8% of the insurance plans essentially amounts over the next 20 years (to) essentially getting rid of the exclusion for employer-sponsored plans."*

Troy and Wilson conclude that the excise tax will affect an increasing number of workers who don't have top-flight health insurance. By 2031 the cost of the *average* family health-care plan is expected to hit the excise-tax threshold. That means the *average* family will be impacted by the 40% tax. They say the creeping reach of this tax is reminiscent of the Alternative Minimum Tax, which was originally designed to hit only the wealthiest taxpayers but now nails the middle class.

This deception of the American people allowed President Obama and his supporters to falsely claim that ObamaCare wouldn't increase taxes on the middle class, a repeated promise made by Obama in his election campaign and in the debate of the new healthcare law. In 2008, presidential candidate Obama vowed:

"I can make a firm pledge. Under my plan, no family making less than $250,000 a year will see any form of tax increase. Not your income tax, not your payroll tax, not your capital gains taxes, not any of your taxes."

Yet, as we have seen in the study above, the tax clearly affects middle-income Americans, and especially unionized industrial workers. This latter group successfully lobbied for a delay of the tax until 2018, but have since discovered the impact is being felt already as they negotiate future labor contracts.

In the presidential campaign of 2008, Republican presidential candidate John McCain put forth a plan for universal coverage health insurance that involved replacing the tax exclusion for employer-sponsored coverage with a universal tax credit that the uninsured could use to purchase health insurance. This transparent elimination of the tax exclusion was excoriated by candidate Obama:

"So here's John McCain's radical plan in a nutshell: he taxes health care benefits for the first time in history. I don't think that's right. . . I reject the tired old debate that says we have to choose between two extremes: government-run health care with higher taxes. . . or insurance companies without rules denying people coverage."

In light of the recent revelations of Jonathan Gruber, healthcare analyst Avik Roy raises an interesting question:

"Was Senator Obama one of the "stupid" American voters with a "lack of economic understanding"? Or was Obama knowledgably, and disingenuously, attacking a feature of Senator McCain's proposal that he later adapted for his own?"

Income Redistribution

Roy goes on to discuss Gruber's comments on the lack of transparency by conceding the tactic worked:

"To a large degree, the tactic of opacity worked. Not only did ObamaCare get passed, but its complex system of cross-subsidies attracted less notice on the Right than did the law's tax hikes and spending increases. But what progressives figured out – and conservatives are just learning – is that government regulation of health insurance can serve as yet another way to redistribute money from one group to another."

He analyzed how the law's health insurance regulations affect people of different ages and genders and found significant impact – especially on young people. For most of the country, young people who shop for coverage on their own have far steeper gross insurance costs under ObamaCare than they did before.

For example, in Louisiana, the underlying cost of insurance increased by 108 percent for 27 year-old men, and 46 percent for 27 year-old women. This is not considered a tax increase by usual terminology but the impact is still the same. For the 27 year-old facing a much more expensive health insurance premium, the effect is the same as a tax increase.

The reason for this increase is that ObamaCare premium pricing is based on what is known as "age-based community rating." Prior to ObamaCare, insurance companies determined premiums based on age, pre-existing medical conditions, geographic location, past expenses, and a variety of other variables. This is called "actuarial rating" and is the most accurate way to predict the cost of providing healthcare benefits.

But ObamaCare insists insurance companies accept everyone regardless of pre-existing medical conditions and only allows them to use age, history of tobacco usage, and geographic location in determining prices. Furthermore, instead of six levels of premium pricing they are only allowed to use three. The result is healthy people pay more than the actual cost of healthcare benefits and sick people pay less.

Figure 1 shows an example taken from the web site for Louisiana. In comparison, the cost of the insurance premium for a healthy 27 year-old male went up by 108 percent while the cost for a 64 year-old rose by only 38 percent. In real dollars, the 64 year-old is still paying more, but the disproportional increase for the 27 year-old is actually a subsidy for the older patient.

What is the real impact of changing from a 6:1 actuarial pricing system, as we experienced before ObamaCare, to the 3:1 age-based community rating we have now? This is illustrated well in Figure 2:

In the first column on the left we see the price for 6:1 actuarial rating. The price of the premium for the youngest insured is $800 and for the oldest is $4800, or six times higher. In the second column we see age-based rating and a 3:1 ratio. The price for the youngest is now $1400 (a 75% increase) and for the oldest it is now $4200 (a 13% *decrease*).

But with the impact of *adverse selection*, which occurs when the youngest people recognize the poor value of their plan and drop out of the program, the prices increase for everyone. In the third column the new prices emerge after calculating the impact of adverse selection. Now the youngest pay $1633 (a 17% further increase) and the oldest pay $4900 (a 17% increase from the middle column but only a 2% increase from the original price). The youngest are now paying 104% of the original price of $800.

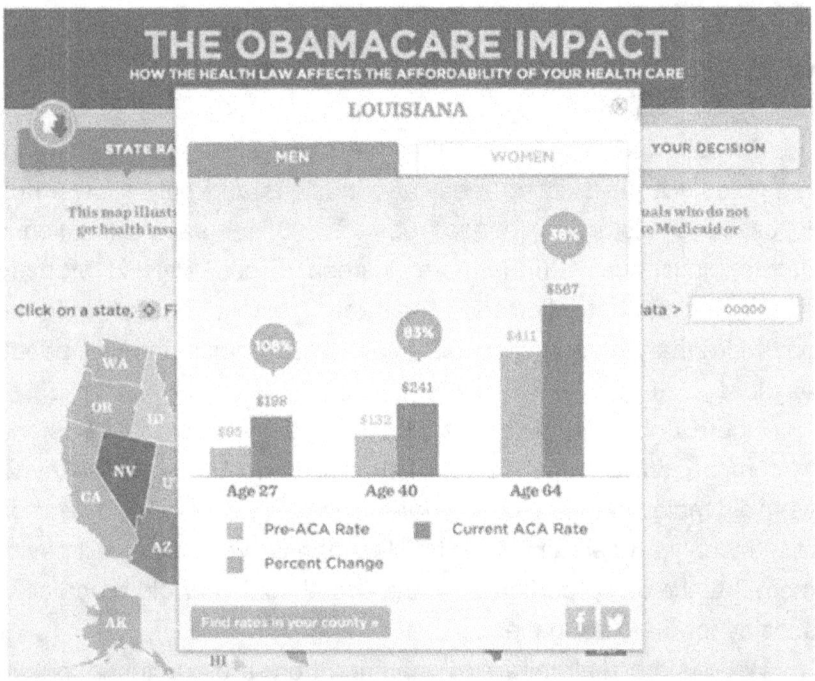

Figure 1 - Comparison of insurance premium prices by age and gender.

The illustration shows how wealth is redistributed from one group to another. In this case, the redistribution is from young people to old people – ironically from an age-group likely to have less money to an age-group likely to have more money. In this way ObamaCare not only hides its redistributive design but imperfectly transfers wealth from one group to another. Young people are harmed the most – even though they were largely responsible for electing President Obama.

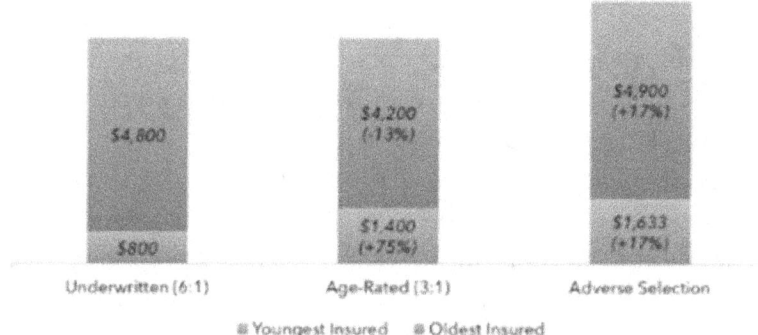

Underwritten (6:1)   Age-Rated (3:1)   Adverse Selection

■ Youngest Insured   ■ Oldest Insured

Forcing the young to pay more drives costs up for everyone. The average 64-year-old consumes six times as much health care, in dollar value, as the average 21-year-old. Hence, in an underwritten (i.e., actuarially priced) insurance market, insurance premiums for 64-year-olds are roughly six times as costly as those for 21-year-olds. Under the ACA, policies are age-rated, i.e., insurers cannot charge their oldest policyholders more than three times what they charge their youngest customers. If every customer remains in the insurance market, this has the net effect of increasing premiums for 21-year-olds by 75 percent, and reducing them for 64-year-olds by 13 percent. However, if half of the 21-year-olds recognize this development as a bad deal for them, and drop out of the market, adverse selection ensues, driving up the average health care consumption per policyholder, thereby driving premiums up for everyone, including the 64-year-olds who were supposed to benefit from 3:1 age rating. In an attempt to mitigate this problem, the ACA includes an individual mandate forcing most young people to purchase government-certified insurance.

<u>Figure 2</u> - Aged-based community rating and Adverse Selection.

Once again, Gruber admits the duplicity of the Obama administration. On the videotapes he concedes:

"If you had a law which . . . made explicit that healthy people pay in and sick people get money, it would not have passed."

Manipulation of the CBO

Gruber's tapes repeatedly document the deliberate deception, not only of the American people, but also of the Congressional Budget Office (CBO). They used a decade of taxes to fund merely six years of insurance subsidies (government expenses) so that the CBO scoring of the bill would be budget neutral. This allowed President Obama to falsely claim the bill *"would not increase the deficit by a dime."*

But Gruber also identifies a special liberal manipulation: CBO's policy reversal to not count the Individual Mandate to buy insurance as an explicit component of the federal budget. The Editorial Board of *The Wall Street Journal* points out the significance of this manipulation:

"In 1994, then CBO chief Robert Reischauer reasonably determined that if the government forces people to buy a product by law, then those transactions no longer belong to the private economy but to the U.S. balance sheet. The CBO's face-melting cost estimate helped to kill HillaryCare.

The CBO director responsible for this switcheroo that moved much of ObamaCare's real spending off the books was Peter Orszag, who went on to become Mr. Obama's budget director. Mr. Orszag nonetheless assailed CBO during the debate for not giving him enough credit for the law's phantom 'savings'."

Thus Gruber, with the help of Peter Orszag, found a way to avoid the pitfall of the Clinton administration that helped to sink HillaryCare.

The Wall Street Journal goes on to point out that in an earlier Gruber tape before an audience at Holy Cross University in 2010, he lamented ObamaCare *"is 90% health insurance coverage and 10% about cost control, (but) all you ever hear people talk about is cost control. How it's going to lower the cost of health care, that's all they talk about. Why? Because that's what people want to hear about because a majority of Americans care about health-care costs."*

They warn that Mr. Gruber's honesty is another warning that the budget rules are rigged to expand government and hide the true cost of entitlements. CBO scores aren't unambiguous facts but are guesses about the future, biased by the Keynesian assumptions and models its political masters in Congress instruct it to use.

Democrats Run From Gruber

The White House and leading Democrats like House Minority Leader Nancy Pelosi have tried to distance themselves from Gruber's remarks by denying any association with him. When asked to comment on Gruber's remarks, Pelosi said this:

"I don't know who he is. He didn't write our bill."

Yet in 2009 she specifically cited Gruber's analysis of the health care bill in the debate before passage of the law. Videotape of Pelosi confirms her support of him in which she uses his analysis as evidence of the bill's credibility. His work was quoted and linked on her website at that time.

President Obama also tried to distance himself from Gruber's remarks. At a press conference while traveling in Burma, Obama responded to a question about Gruber's comments by saying:

"The fact that some advisor who never worked on our staff expressed an opinion that I completely disagree with in terms of the voters, is no reflection of the actual process that was run."

Yet the public record of the White House confirms, and Gruber's public statements agree, that Gruber visited the White House on 19 separate occasions during the debate and design of ObamaCare and was paid nearly $400,000 by HHS for his expertise and consultations. More videotape documents President Obama's support of Gruber and his analysis of the new law and holds him out as the world recognized expert on healthcare economics that he is. An investigation by Fox News revealed Gruber has been paid $5.9 million by HHS and multiple states in the last 15 years for analysis and consultation on the development of healthcare policies.

Even Gruber, for all the credit he has been given for honesty, tried to distance himself from his own remarks:

"The comments in the video were made at an academic conference," Gruber told MSNBC. *"I was speaking off the cuff. I basically spoke inappropriately. I regret having made those comments."*

That might have sufficed if there were only one video. But with the emergence of multiple videos that revealed the same essential views, even Gruber could not escape the candor and ramifications of his comments.

The credibility of Gruber was never in question *before* the passage of ObamaCare. He has helped in the development of healthcare systems in Massachusetts, California, Connecticut, Delaware, Kansas, Minnesota, Oregon, Wisconsin and Wyoming. He was heralded by the liberal media including *The New York Times'* Catherine Rampell who wrote this in 2012:

"Mr. Gruber has spent decades modeling the intricacies of the health care ecosystem, which involves making predictions about how new laws will play out based on past experience and economic theory. It is his research that convinced the Obama administration that health care reform could not work without requiring everyone to buy insurance."

He also has the respect of other healthcare economists including Harvard's David Cutler, another architect of ObamaCare. Although Cutler disagreed with Gruber regarding the importance of the individual mandate, he nevertheless acknowledged his expertise in the following statement:

"He's brought a level of science to an issue that would otherwise be just opinion. He's really the only person who has been doing all this careful modeling for so long. He's the only person you can go to for that kind of thing, which is why the White House reached out to him in the first place."

The Insurance Subsidies Issue

Perhaps the most significant of the Gruber tapes are those that document the intent of Congress when they passed the healthcare law with regard to eligibility for subsidies of health insurance premiums.

As discussed earlier in Chapter Two, at issue is the government's interpretation of the wording of the law regarding who would receive subsidies. The actual wording of the statute is subsidies are available for those who purchase premiums on "*exchanges established by the State.*" When only 16 states chose to establish their own exchanges, the Obama administration directed the IRS to allow subsidies also for those purchasing premiums on the federal exchange. They argue this was the original intent of Congress.

But Gruber's tapes tell a different story:

"If you're a state and you don't set up an exchange, that means your citizens don't get their tax credits. I hope that that's a blatant enough political reality that states will get their act together and realize there are billions of dollars at stake here in setting up these exchanges."

Gruber's comments as one of the original architects of the law clearly establish the government understood the law limited subsidies to state exchanges. It was the intent of the law to preserve the sovereignty of the states while pressuring them to comply with the government's desire for all states to establish their own exchanges. When the states objected to this pressure, and chose not to establish their own exchanges, the Obama administration decided to reinterpret the law.

This issue will be decided by the Supreme Court within the next term of the court which ends June 30, 2015. The High Court accepted the appeal of *King v. Burwell* on this issue and oral arguments were already heard on March 4, 2015. If the Supreme Court upholds the law as written, it could bring about a radical change in the law or perhaps its repeal. Once again, the videotapes of Jonathan Gruber have given us candor about this healthcare legislation that has been wholly lacking from the Obama administration.

Syndicated columnist Charles Krauthammer summarizes the importance of these Gruber videotapes:

"It's refreshing that "the most transparent administration in history," as this administration fancies itself, should finally display candor about its signature act of social change. Inadvertently, of course. But now we know what lay behind Obama's smooth reassurances – the arrogance of an academic liberalism that rules in the name of a citizenry it mocks, disdains, and deliberately, contemptuously deceives."

15

The Impact of the Mid-term Elections

"Barack Obama once said that he wanted to be as consequential in his own way as Ronald Reagan was. He is in this sense: he is the greatest builder of the Republican Party since Ronald Reagan."
Syndicated columnist George Will - 11/19/14

A recent advertisement slogan reminds us *"life comes at you fast."* In 2008 Barack Obama was swept into office as the 44th President of the United States on a wave of Democratic optimism. Running on a campaign of "Hope and Change" he won nearly 53% of the vote, the largest percentage of the popular vote for a Democrat in nearly half a century. He won 365 electoral votes to John McCain's 173. Democrats were ascendant and nothing seemed unachievable in their quest to enact their liberal agenda.

But as I write these words in November 2014, for the second time in four years, Republicans have ridden an equally impressive wave to capture control of both Houses of Congress in the mid-term elections. There have always been ups and downs in the fortunes of political parties, but rarely have we seen such a dramatic change in so little time.

The principle explanation for this dramatic change of political fortunes can be attributed to President Obama's "signature legislation" – *ObamaCare.*

A careful analysis of the 2010 mid-term elections conducted by five political scientists revealed at least 25 members of Congress lost their seats in Congress because they voted for ObamaCare. Such a sophisticated analysis took 17 months after that election was over, so it's much too soon to report on the impact of the 2014 mid-term elections. But the evidence is quickly mounting that ObamaCare was also responsible for the huge victories Republicans enjoyed in 2014.

Chris Conover, writing in *Forbes,* suggests five reasons ObamaCare played an important role in this election:

- *First - Public opposition to the law actually was slightly stronger in November 2014 than it was in November 2010.* The Real Clear Politics average of polls can be seen in Figure 1 below:

Polling Data					
Poll	Date	Sample	For/Favor	Against/Oppose	Spread
RCP Average	10/8 - 11/13	--	37.7	51.6	Against/Oppose +13.9
Gallup	11/6 - 11/9	828 A	37	56	Against/Oppose +19
Rasmussen Reports	11/12 - 11/13	1000 LV	40	50	Against/Oppose +10
Pew Research	11/6 - 11/9	1353 A	45	51	Against/Oppose +6
CBS News	10/23 - 10/27	1269 A	36	55	Against/Oppose +19
Associated Press/GfK	10/16 - 10/20	968 LV	31	48	Against/Oppose +17
FOX News	10/12 - 10/14	831 LV	39	53	Against/Oppose +14
NBC News/Wall St. Jrnl	10/8 - 10/12	1000 RV	36	48	Against/Oppose +12
All Public Approval of Health Care Law Polling Data					

Figure 1: Real Clear Politics average of polls and the polls separately.

The RCP average shows nearly 52 percent opposed with 38 percent in favor of ObamaCare. The Gallup poll shows as much as a 19-point difference with 56 percent opposed and 37 percent in favor. The historical trend of ObamaCare disapproval can be traced on the graph illustrated below in Figure 2.

Figure 2 clearly shows the trend is getting worse for ObamaCare. Rather than growing in popularity, as then-House Majority Leader Nancy Pelosi famously predicted, ObamaCare is gaining opposition. Despite Paul Krugman's claims to the contrary, the law is failing (Introduction).

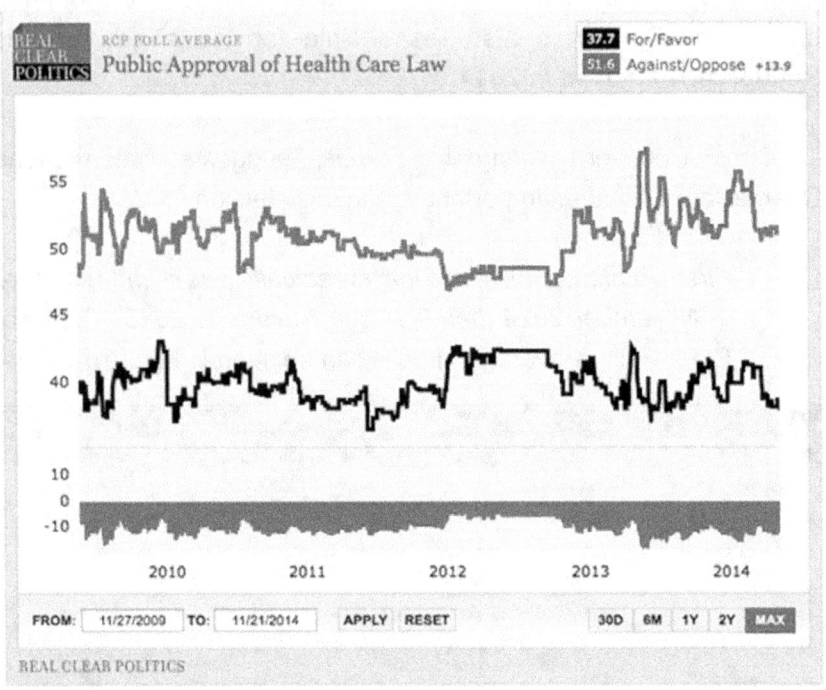

Figure 2: Real Clear Politics average from 11/27/09 to 11/21/14. The bottom of the three graphics shows the difference between the two averages 13.9 % (oppose). (Note the difference has never been in favor of the law.)

- *Second – ObamaCare is a deciding issue among those voters who are most passionate about voting.* A recent survey conducted by Public Opinion Strategies (POS) for Independent Women's Voice revealed this before the election.

- *Third – Exit polls confirmed this survey with 49% indicating they thought ObamCare "went too far."* (25% thought it did not go far enough; 21% thought it was "about right.") Of those who thought the law went too far, 84% voted Republican and only 14% voted Democrat.
- *Fourth – Every new Republican member of the U.S. Senate promised to "repeal and replace ObamaCare."* This issue probably was the swing issue in closely contested races in North Carolina, where Senator Kay Hagan defended the law, and Virginia, where Republican Ed Gillespie nearly pulled off the upset of the night by offering a credible, detailed alternative to ObamaCare.
- *Fifth – Even with one election undecided, Republicans now hold 31 governorships, just one less than their historical record.* The campaign pledges of Republicans regarding Medicaid expansion seem to have been crucial. Even *The New York Times* concedes: *"the election results did not replace any expansion-opposing governors with expansion advocates."*

How big was the Republican victory?

The last Senatorial race of 2014 was decided on December 8 when incumbent Democratic Senator Mary Landrieu of Louisiana was defeated by Republican Congressman Bill Cassidy. That gives Republicans 54 seats in the Senate compared to 44 for Democrats and 2 for Independents. In the House of Representatives, Republicans increased their majority margin from 233 v. 199 before the election to 246 v. 188 (1 undecided) after the election. Republicans gained 9 seats in the Senate and 13 in the House.

The Republican wave of this election has achieved historical gains. The GOP now controls 68 out of 99 partisan state legislative chambers – the highest in the history of the party. They have 31 governorships with Democrats holding 17, Independents 1, and one undecided. They have majorities in both the House of Representatives and the Senate for the first time since the 109th Congress of President

George W. Bush and the largest margin of control since 1929. As George Will said in the opening quote to this chapter, *"Barack Obama is the greatest builder of the Republican Party since Ronald Reagan."*

Figure 3 illustrates the party dominance of Congress since the post-Civil War era of 1869. The last Congress so well represented by Republicans dates all the way back to the 71st Congress of 1929. Since then Congress has been largely dominated by the Democrats. It is ironic that Barack Obama, the man many thought would lead to a permanent Democratic majority, has restored the Republican control of Congress.

Party dominance in Congress

The majority of each chamber of Congress as a percentage of membership, by party and combined.

SENATE   HOUSE

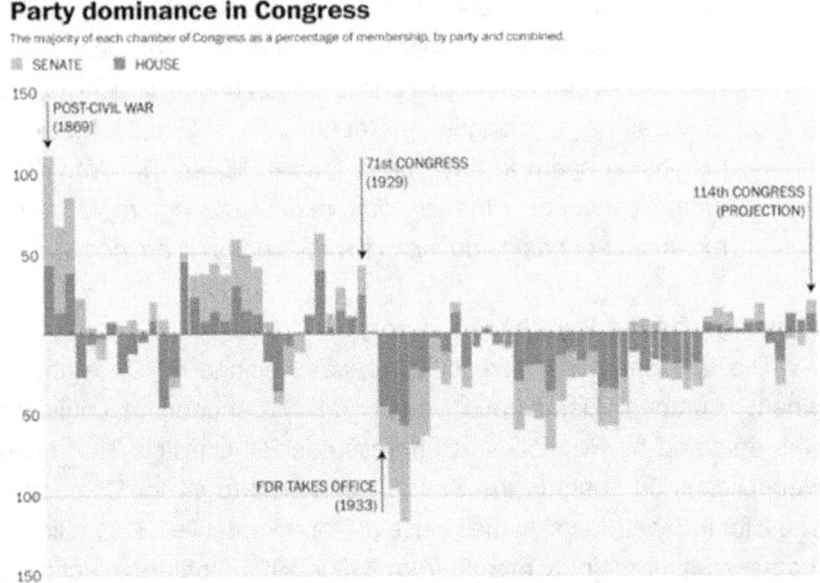

Figure 3 – History of political party dominance in Congress 1869 – 2014.

How have Democrats fared who voted for ObamaCare?

ObamaCare was passed without a single Republican vote in either houses of Congress. How have Democrats fared who voted for this legislation?

In the Senate, where 60 Democratic votes were necessary to pass the Affordable Care Act, only 30 of those Democrats will remain in office with the new Congress in January 2015. Three of the ObamaCare 60 died in office, while 19 declined to run for re-election. Some left to take other jobs in the administration such as John Kerry, who became Secretary of State.

But others could read the writing on the wall and declined to run for re-election. These include Chris Dodd (CT), Jim Webb (VA), Ben Nelson (NE), Jay Rockefeller (WV), Max Baucus (MT), Tim Johnson (SD) and Jay Dorgan (ND). The rest ran for re-election and were handed a pink slip by the voters. These include Ms. Landrieu (LA), Mark Begich (AK), Kay Hagan (NC), Blanche Lincoln and Mark Pryor (AR), Russ Feingold (WI) and Mark Udall (C0). Republican cross-over Arlen Specter left the GOP to vote for ObamaCare and then lost the Democratic primary in his re-election bid to Joe Sestak, who lost to Republican Pat Toomey.

Democrats never saw this coming. President Obama told Democrats at a March 2010 pep rally that he knew they faced "*a tough vote*" but was "*actually confident*" that "*it will end up being the smart thing to do politically because I believe that good policy is good politics.*" Even New York Senator Chuck Schumer claimed on NBC's "Meet the Press" that "*by November those who voted for health care will find it an asset, those who voted against it will find it a liability.*"

These words are particularly remarkable in hindsight since Senator Schumer recently recanted this assessment, calling ObamaCare a disaster for the Democratic Party. *The Wall Street Journal* editorial board sums it up well:

"*As it happens, the law has been nearly as politically catastrophic for Democrats as Watergate was for Republicans. . . Such is the political price Democrats are paying for ignoring voters and passing what we called at the time the worst law since FDR's national Industrial Recovery Act and the Smoot-Hawley tariff.*"

How should Republicans respond?

With control of both the House and the Senate, Republicans are poised to make substantial changes in ObamaCare. Democrats, however, still control the White House and President Obama will be loath to accept Republican attempts to repeal or even modify the law. Outright repeal is highly unlikely as long as President Obama is in office since Republicans will have great difficulty obtaining sufficient Democratic support to nullify an Obama veto.

Therefore, Republicans should look to modify or repeal those parts of the law that already enjoy bipartisan support. In the days since the mid-term elections, many political pundits have expressed their views on what changes Republicans should seek. Here is a review of some of these recommendations:

Avik Roy – Forbes

Avik Roy, Fellow at The Manhattan Institute and healthcare blogger for *Forbes,* proposes seven ObamaCare bills the GOP should pass in 2015. There is a budget impact of each of these changes and is estimated below each:

- **Give states more flexibility and authority** – Return insurance regulation to the province of the states – where it has usually been in the past. Congress should restore as much of that state-based regulatory authority as possible. This should include giving states the flexibility to run their Medicaid programs in a way to fit their circumstances.
  - o *Fiscal surplus – Depends on specifics*
- **Liberalize ObamaCare's insurance exchanges** – Republicans could pass laws giving insurers more flexibility to offer affordable products – like generic drugs whenever possible. Some Democrats have supported the idea of offering "copper" plans that would have higher deductibles – and lower premiums – than the costlier plans on ObamaCare's

exchanges. Such plans could significantly reduce the cost of ObamaCare-based health insurance.

  o *Fiscal surplus - $1 billion a year*

- **Repeal ObamaCare's Employer Mandate** – Even liberal writers like Jonathan Cohn of *The New Republic* and Timothy Jost of *Health Affairs Blog* support this idea. This mandate has caused economic chaos by encouraging businesses to limit employees to 29-hour work weeks and companies to 49 employees. Several independent analyses, most notably one from the CBO, have indicated that repealing the mandate would have a negligible effect on the number of Americans with health insurance.

  o *Fiscal cost - $10 billion a year*

- **Repeal ObamaCare's medical device, pharmaceutical, and health insurance excise taxes** – This is the "low hanging fruit" bill since they already have wide bipartisan support. The tax of 2.3% on all medical devices has had a huge negative impact on the medical device industry, and is stifling medical innovation (see Chapter Ten). These companies are mostly located in blue states – those controlled by Democratic senators. These include the largest medical device companies such as **Johnson & Johnson** (New Jersey), **Medtronic** (Minnesota), **Baxter** (Illinois), **Stryker** (Michigan), **Boston Scientific** (Massachusetts) and **St. Jude** (Minnesota). That explains why some of the most liberal Democratic senators, whose voting records support President Obama more than 90% of the time, are willing to repeal this tax. This group includes Senators Elizabeth Warren (MA), Amy Klobuchar and Al Franken (MN).

  o *Fiscal cost - $10 billion a year*

- **Accelerate or modify ObamaCare's Cadillac tax** – This tax is intended to roll back the tax exclusion for employer-sponsored health insurance (see Chapter 14). Republicans could use enhancements of the Cadillac tax, or wholesale modifications of it, to fund the repeal of ObamaCare's employer mandate and/ or excise taxes. For example, Congress could move the Cadillac tax forward one year. They could eliminate some of the special-interest exemptions (unions) Democrats inserted into the bill. They could modify the way in which the Cadillac tax's threshold increases over time.

- o *Fiscal surplus – Depends on specifics*

- **Repeal ObamaCare's Individual Mandate and age-rating mandate** – ObamaCare includes an Individual Mandate forcing most Americans to purchase government-approved health insurance. That mandate exists, in large part, because ObamaCare drives up the underlying cost of individually-purchased health insurance for young people (Chapter 14). Roy recommends repealing the Individual Mandate *and* the age-based community rating provisions to allow the insurance market to continue to function. This may reduce the number of insured Americans but would have positive budgetary effects. The CBO has projected that repealing the mandate would reduce the deficit by approximately $30 billion a year, which would help to fund other ObamaCare changes.

- o *Fiscal surplus - $30 billion a year*

- **Force the CBO to post its fiscal models online** – Some have called the CBO the Supreme Court of U.S. fiscal policy. But the CBO, and its companion organization the Joint Committee on Taxation, do not disclose the methods they use to come up with projections of the fiscal effects of proposed legislation. This is unacceptable in the 21st century. The CBO has admitted that it does not have the tools to properly model private-sector approaches to covering the uninsured. Roy believes this change is almost certainly the single most important thing that Republicans could do to improve the likelihood of future entitlement reform.

Scott Gottlieb – Forbes

Scott Gottlieb, another *Forbes* contributor, fellow at *The American Enterprise Institute,* and a physician, has his own laundry list of ideas for Republican changes of ObamaCare. There is some overlap with the list of Avik Roy:

- *Medical devices tax*
- *More state flexibility on Medicaid*
- *More flexibility on state-run exchanges*
- *Eliminate the Individual Mandate*
- *Eliminate the Employer Mandate*
- **Repeal the 30-hour definition of full-time work** –This is strangling the job market by forcing employers to keep people under a 30 hour work week to avoid paying health insurance benefits.
- **Repeal the Independent Payment Advisory Board (IPAB)** – Although IPAB has had no real effect yet, the potential for abuse of seniors by arbitrary cuts to Medicare is huge and there is no accountability in the law (Chapter 13).
- **Extend the grandfathering of health plans indefinitely** - This would actually fulfill Obama's famously broken promise, "If you like your plan you can keep your plan."
- **Change the subsidy structure to lower the income threshold** – Currently subsidies are available up to 400% of the Federal Poverty Level (FPL). Use the money saved to pay for other desired changes. Let wealthier families have the option of buying more affordable plans while taxpayers subsidize generously those who are truly priced out of the market.

John R. Graham and Devon Herrick – National Center for Policy Analysis

John R. Graham and Devon Herrick, healthcare analysts at The National Center for Policy Analysis, have their own ideas on how

Republicans should proceed to improve ObamaCare. They agree that ObamaCare cannot be repealed before 2017 but there are many ways Republicans can begin to improve the law. Like those we have read above they agree with the following ideas:

- *Repeal the medical devices tax*
- *Offer "copper" plans with high deductibles*
- *Greater flexibility in Medicaid programs – Wisconsin model*
- *Greater control of Medicare Part D plans to prevent fraud*

But they differ with others, especially with regard to the insurance exchanges. Unlike Avik Roy, they want to eliminate the insurance exchanges. They prefer to use insurance agents, online or in-person, without going through an exchange. The list of changes they would make includes:

- **Eliminate the insurance exchanges**
- **Eliminate the insurance bailout provisions**
- **Shrink the Medicaid expansion**
- **Reduce the power of the FDA to prevent experimental therapies – "Right to Try"**

James C. Capretta – Ethics and Public Policy Center

James C. Capretta, senior fellow at the Ethics and Public Policy Center and a visiting fellow at the American Enterprise Institute, has written extensively on ObamaCare and especially regarding conservative alternatives. He has some advice for Republicans now that they control both houses of Congress:

- **Keep your eyes on 2016** – A Republican Congress cannot repeal ObamaCare while president Obama is in office. This will only happen should Republicans prevail in the 2016 presidential election. Therefore, he says Republicans should ask themselves before every decision: "Will this help or hurt our nominee in 2016?"

- *Pick your targets carefully* – He suggests allowing anyone who wanted to stay in the insurance plan they had before ObamaCare keep their plan. They could also limit subsidies for insurers participating in the ObamaCare exchanges and eliminate the tax people must pay for going uninsured (the Individual Mandate). He also recommends repealing the Employer Mandate, which should have bipartisan support. He also favors repeal of IPAB.

- *Use reconciliation strategically* – This legislative maneuver, which was used by the Democrats to push through ObamaCare without the usual 60 votes, should be avoided as a means to push through full repeal. This would only further divide the country and the president would veto the move anyway. He does believe it would be useful to advance pieces of a repeal-and-replace strategy. The key is to find changes that can divide the coalition in support of ObamaCare and thus put pressure on the president to sign the legislation.

- *Be realistic about replace* – A Republican plan to replace ObamaCare needs to provide secure insurance for the sick and put affordable coverage within the financial reach of all Americans. It should not disrupt the employer coverage that most middle-income families have and like. These principles can form the basis of a practical strategy to replace ObamaCare, and Republicans would be wise to rally around them to set the stage for the next presidential administration.

What else should be done?

Conspicuous by its absence are any recommendations to fix the gap that currently exists between Medicaid coverage and subsidies on the insurance exchanges. This "**Medicaid gap**" coverage exists in those states where the offer to expand Medicaid was declined by the state.

ObamaCare offers to pay 100% of the cost of Medicaid expansion through 2016 and 90% thereafter, at least until 2020. Then it sets the upper limit of Medicaid expansion eligibility, 138% of FPL, as the lower limit of eligibility for subsidies to purchase private insurance on the exchanges.

However, if you live in a state that decided not to expand Medicaid, then you are eligible for Medicaid by the old definitions, whatever that is in your state. For example, if you live in Alabama, where Medicaid eligibility is 25% of FPL, and you earn more than 25% of FPL – but less than 138% of FPL – you earn *too much* to be eligible for Medicaid and *too little* to be eligible for a subsidy to purchase private insurance. These people are the truly unfortunate.

This problem could be fixed easily by making anyone ineligible for Medicaid eligible for the same subsidies as those earning 139% of FPL. This gap in coverage was probably never intended because those writing this legislation thought all the states would welcome Medicaid expansion. But they arrogantly assumed that states would welcome this Medicaid expansion, despite the fact that the federal government is over $17 Trillion in debt. Governors have to balance their budgets even though the federal government does not.

People Forced Onto Medicaid

There is another related problem with ObamaCare. The expansion of Medicaid eligibility has forced some families onto Medicaid that don't want to be there. If you earn 125% of FPL, in most states, you were purchasing private healthcare insurance before ObamaCare. But now with the expanded eligibility of Medicaid, if your state accepted the expansion, you may be forced onto Medicaid even though you want to purchase private insurance.

According to a new study from the Heritage Foundation, the number of insured Americans increased by 8.5 million. However, 71% of the increase comes from expansion of the rolls of Medicaid. According to the study:

- Individual market enrollment – meaning enrollment in health insurance plans both on and off of the exchanges – rose by more than 6.2 million.
- Employer-sponsored private plan enrollment, however, fell by almost 3.8 million, offsetting 61% of the increase in health insurance coverage in the individual market.
- Enrollment in Medicaid grew by more than 5.7 million in the states that expanded Medicaid. In the states that did not, enrollment in the government health care program grew by more than 355,000.

Since half the states rejected the ObamaCare offer to expand Medicaid in their states, this high percentage of new enrollees in Medicaid is surprising. But a testimonial from a general surgeon in Arizona explains what is happening.

Dr. Jeffrey A. Singer, from Phoenix, writes in *The Wall Street Journal* that Medicaid is stealing patients from private insurance – without their consent. He tells of many of his patients who were forced into Medicaid when they tried to renew their private health insurance on the exchanges. He says this experience is not unusual and a recent Boston University/Harvard Medical School study backs him up.

The study reveals that up to 80% of people participating in ObamaCare's Medicaid expansion have been shifted off their private insurance. These patients' plans did not meet ACA requirements and were therefore cancelled. Despite the fact that the patients liked their plans, they were forced into accepting Medicaid because that was all that Healthcare.gov offered them.

Therefore, many of those newly enrolled in Medicaid are *not newly insured*. They lost private health insurance due to ObamaCare and now can only be insured by Medicaid. Now they're trapped in an inferior health care system. (Chapter Four)

Today only 45% of doctors are accepting new Medicaid patients, according to a recent survey by the healthcare company Merritt Hawkins. This number has dropped from 55% in the past five years.

In some cities – Dallas and Minneapolis, for example – as few as 23% of doctors are seeing new Medicaid patients. This means longer waiting times to get appointments for primary care – and even longer waiting times to see a specialist. This problem will only get worse with the increase of the number of Medicaid patients seeking care from a declining number of providers. Yet ObamaCare is forcing many people into Medicaid that formerly enjoyed private health insurance.

The authors of the Heritage Foundation study, Edmund Haislmaier and Drew Gonshorowski, conclude: *"The inescapable conclusion is that, at least when it comes to covering the uninsured, ObamaCare so far is mainly a simple expansion of Medicaid."*

The goal for ObamaCare was to solve the problem of uninsured Americans by providing insurance for those previously uninsured. Forcing people *with* private health insurance onto Medicaid is no solution at all.

Therefore, Republicans should try to keep people in private insurance as much as possible, especially those who never wanted to be on Medicaid in the first place.

A Two-Step Approach to Reform

In summary, there are many proposals listed above to reform ObamaCare until the law can be fully repealed and replaced with a conservative, market-based alternative (Chapter Twelve). But until then, a two-step approach is advocated by several of the writers mentioned above.

This two-step approach calls for strategic thinking. The first step is a systematic series of votes – perhaps one a month beginning shortly after the new Congress is sworn in January 2015. The wide bipartisan support for elimination of the medical devices tax should be the first order of business and then move on from there to other harder issues such as eliminating the Individual Mandate and the Employer Mandate.

Even if President Obama vetoes some of these bills, the Republicans will have shown what they stand for and what the

American people can expect if they elect a Republican president in 2016. It would be best if this strategy is well-established before June 2015 when the Supreme Court will rule on *King v. Burwell* (Chapter Two). Chris Conover explains the importance of this strategy:

"A decision to invalidate federal subsidies on federally-run Exchanges will offer Republicans the maximum possible leverage to get the president and Democrats in Congress to a more reasonable accommodation on where health reform should be headed going forward. It positions Republicans to offer a "grand bargain" of sorts, i.e., an agreement to fix the subsidy language if and only if other major reforms such as eliminating the individual mandate are included."

Regardless of the president's reaction, pro or con, Republicans will gain politically by their initiative. They will either gain immediately by the improvements to the law or they will gain politically in the run-up to the 2016 elections because the president doubles-down on his obstinate refusal to improve a law opposed by a majority of Americans.

The second part of the strategy is to use the next two years to lay the groundwork – through congressional hearings, etc. – for a comprehensive approach to reforming or replacing ObamaCare. Eventually Republicans should rally around a single plan; but until then, they need only put the essential elements of an improved alternative on the table for open discussion. They *do need*, however, to demonstrate to the American electorate that they have a better plan than ObamaCare and they will implement it, given a Republican president in 2016.

Conclusions

"Americans are flagrantly ill-informed . . . a nation of dodos."
Joe Klein, *Time* magazine, 1/25/10

Sadly, most Americans are uninformed. It has been my purpose in writing this book to make a small dent in this problem so indelicately described above by *Times* magazine columnist Joe Klein. The fate of our Republic rests on the shoulders of an informed electorate.

This opinion is not original. In fact it was fundamental to the Founding Fathers including Thomas Jefferson and James Madison:

*"I know no safe depositary of the ultimate powers of the society but the people themselves; and if we think them not enlightened enough to exercise their control with a wholesome discretion, the remedy is not to take it from them, but to inform their discretion by education. This is the true corrective of abuses of constitutional power." --****Thomas Jefferson*** *to William C. Jarvis, 1820. ME 15:278*

*"Above all things I hope the education of the common people will be attended to, convinced that on their good sense we may rely with the most security for the preservation of a due degree of liberty." --****Thomas Jefferson*** *to James Madison, 1787. Madison Version FE 4:480*

"Whenever the people are well-informed, they can be trusted with their own government;... whenever things get so far wrong as

to attract their notice, they may be relied on to set them to rights."
*--**Thomas Jefferson** to Richard Price, 1789. ME 7:253*

"Knowledge will forever govern ignorance, and a people who mean to be their own governors must arm themselves with the power which knowledge gives."
James Madison

"I believe there are more instances of the abridgement of freedom of the people by gradual and silent encroachments by those in power than by violent and sudden usurpations."
James Madison

Many Americans fail to keep themselves informed about their government and the changes that government imposes on their lives. If you are reading this book, you are not one of these Americans. But it is necessary that we all work to keep our fellow citizens informed.

Unlike men such as Jefferson and Madison, many of our current politicians and their enablers believe that only they are capable of making the important decisions that affect the lives of all Americans. We have seen this attitude on harsh display by Jonathan Gruber, Ph.D., the MIT economist discussed in Chapter Fourteen. His attitude is not unique, but is embodied by those sometimes referred to as "the Ruling Class".

The Ruling Class

It has been the dream of the Progressives for over a hundred years to socialize medicine. In my previous book, *The ObamaCare Train Wreck,* I traced the history of the Progressive movement to change our system of health care in order to increase government control and redistribute wealth.

This Progressive movement has carried the banner of both political parties, beginning with Republican President Theodore Roosevelt, but since then, adopting Democratic Party leaders such as President Woodrow Wilson, Franklin D. Roosevelt and Lyndon B. Johnson.

Today, it is President Barack Obama who has finally brought the Progressives their long-sought goal. It is for this reason they fought so hard to pass the Affordable Care Act (ObamaCare), despite the clear indication that a majority of the American people did not support it. Through a series of political back-room maneuvers and Congressional slick tricks, they managed to pass the bill without a single Republican vote.

Why would they insist upon passing legislation that did not have the backing of a majority of the American people?

The answer to this question can be found in a book called *The Ruling Class* by Angelo Codevilla. He defines our country into two groups; not by political parties, but by their self-image and attitudes defined by their educational biases and socioeconomic upbringing.

The first of these is called the **Ruling Class**. This group believes that only those in their "elite" status are qualified to govern the country. Although many are wealthy, it is not their wealth that gives them "ruling class status." Rather it is their educational credentials and their connections to the government.

While they attended the best schools, it is not their academic performances that distinguish them. In fact, many were admitted to these schools not on the basis of their grades but on the basis of their social pedigree. What matters most in Codevilla's words is *"their commitment to fit in."*

Those in the Ruling Class believe it is their duty to make decisions "for the good of the country" that ordinary citizens are incapable of making. This condescending attitude is the hallmark of their class. It justifies their determination to decide what light bulbs we put in our lamps, what food we put on our tables, what toilets we allow in our homes and what fuel we put in our cars.

Ruling Class members do not believe that "all men are created equal." They believe the obvious differences in the talents and abilities of people justify their presumption that "they know what's best for the country." They do not believe in a higher power and in general mock those who do. For this reason they are often known as "secular progressives."

President Barack Obama demonstrated this dismissiveness when he was caught on tape describing his opponents' *"clinging to God and guns"* as a characteristic of inferior Americans. To justify himself he said he was only pointing out "what *everybody* knows is true."

The Country Class

The other group is called the **Country Class.** This heterogeneous group represents most Americans who believe that the Declaration of Independence got it right; that "all men are created equal" means everyone should have equal protections under the law and equal opportunity to pursue the American dream.

They believe they can make their own choices on light bulbs, toilets, food, and fuel to put in their cars, not to mention the amount of water that flows out of their shower nozzle. Most believe in a higher power, and they don't want the government to interfere with their religious liberty that was paid for with the blood of our forefathers. This group represents the large majority of Americans.

The Ruling Class is dismissive of the opinions of the Country Class because they believe in their hearts they are doing a noble thing; determining the future of our country. This explains why the Obama administration dismissed the advice of governors and healthcare professionals in drafting the Affordable Care Act and chose instead to listen to academics like Jonathan Gruber and others of their own class. In so doing they have created a monster that not only will ruin the health care system in this country but will expose the weaknesses of their own ideology.

In his campaign rhetoric of 2008, Barack Obama referred to himself and his followers as *"we are the ones we've been waiting for."* But since those heady days of Obama's rise to power, *reality has taken a different course.*

It is that reality that forms the basis and purpose of this book. Although Obama was able to pass his signature health care legislation, the country's response has been less than enthusiastic. In fact, it has been down right negative. Not once since the passage of the ACA has there been a national poll that showed a majority of Americans favored the new law. At the completion of this book at the end of 2014, the latest Gallop poll showed only 37% of Americans favored Obama's healthcare legislation. Yet those in the Ruling Class, as exemplified by Princeton economist Paul Krugman (see Introduction), still think the law is a success.

In his book *The Revolt Against the Masses,* author Fred Siegel writes of the weaknesses of those who would presume to be best qualified to lead us. Much like Codevilla, he exposes the arrogance of the Ruling Class. Noemie Emery of *The Weekly Standard* writes that Siegel noted,

"They had too much belief in the brilliance of experts, they were completely dismissive of public opinion, and they had a contempt for the great middle class."

This adroitly describes those who drafted ObamaCare – now documented by the videotapes of Jonathan Gruber.

Emery describes the writing of the bill with a familiar metaphor:

"If a camel is a horse designed by a committee, this camel was a 2,801-page non-bestseller filled with labyrinthine riddles that nobody seemed to know how to solve. To insure approximately 18 million out of 300-plus million Americans (they confessed the plan would still leave 20 million uninsured), they proposed to spend trillions on a reengineering of the entire system that would in time cause 80 to 100 million of the currently insured to lose and to seek new insurance."

Rather than rely on the experience of Governors whose state programs demonstrated successful programs to copy, like President Bill Clinton did with the Welfare Reform Act of 1996, Obama chose to look to his fellow elites in the Ruling Class. Emery describes it this way:

"The Affordable Care Act looked for advice to academics, not governors, and proposed the state takeover of an industrial complex responsible for one-sixth of the gross national product based not on what had been proved to work through experience, but on what some intellectuals had guessed might work."

Previous government entitlement programs such as Social Security and Medicare enjoyed bipartisan support. For this reason they remain popular and have become "the third rail" of politics; too dangerous to touch. But ObamaCare was passed without a single Republican vote and remains unpopular by a significant majority. When common sense would have led most people to compromise their plans to gain support, the Obama administration, true to their "Ruling Class" status, doubled-down on their rhetoric and pushed through the unpopular legislation.

But the dream that took a hundred years to fulfill is rapidly becoming a nightmare they wish would go away. Democrats are in denial when they say they are proud of ObamaCare and expect to campaign on its benefits. Democratic leadership like House Minority Leader Nancy Pelosi or Democratic Party Chairman Debbie Wasserman Schultz pushed back when Republicans suggested they had a great campaign issue in ObamaCare, but the results of the November mid-term elections proved the American people sided with the Republicans.

Emery writes that ObamaCare has already terminated the careers of almost 70 national Democrats, given the Republicans' control of 26 states, and brought in a new crew of GOP leaders inspired to fight this new legislation. (And that was before the results of the November elections were known). It has drained President Obama of the political momentum to advance the rest of his liberal agenda leaving him to resort to finding ways, many of them illegal, to go around Congress to accomplish his goals.

Studies Confirm the Failure of ObamaCare

Shortly before publication of this book, several studies revealed the objective evidence that ObamaCare is not working. One year after the end of the first open enrollment period, the failures of this law can now be measured.

John Graham of The National Center for Policy Analysis compared the latest estimates from the Centers for Disease Control and Prevention (CDC) with their survey from a decade ago. He summarizes this comparison:

*"The proportion of people of all ages with a "usual place to go for medical care" was 87.8 percent last year, **the same as it was in 2002-2003**. Further, 5.7 percent reported that they failed to obtain needed medical care due to cost last year, **the same as it was in 2003-2004."***

No difference! Ten years later and despite spending billions on ObamaCare, there is no difference. No improvement in the percentage of people who can regularly receive medical care. No decline in the number who failed to obtain needed medical care. Maybe this is just an isolated finding in one study.

Actually it is not. Another study looked at data last year from 16,000 providers across the country, collected by **AthenaHealth**. This study shows the requests for new appointments just barely edged upward in 2014. The proportion of new patient visits to primary care doctors increased from 22.6 percent in 2013 to 22.9 percent in 2014. (See Figure 1.)

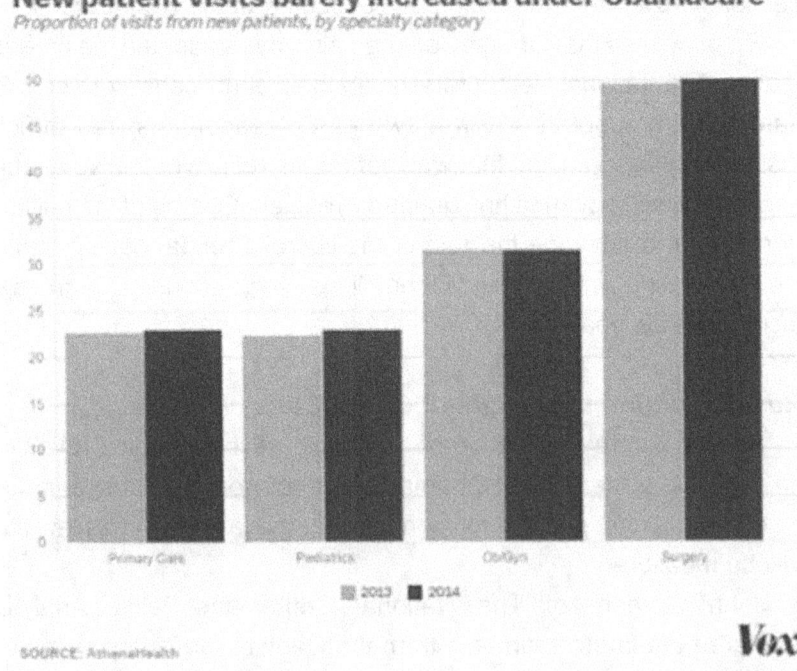

Figure 1 – New patient visits barely increased under ObamaCare.

Further evidence comes from a look at the Massachusetts health reform experience, which was the foundational basis for the architects of ObamaCare. A new study, published in the Boston Medical Journal policy journal, examined hospitalization in Massachusetts for 12 medical conditions that wouldn't normally require hospitalization if a patient has good access to primary care. These are thought to be a good measure of access to healthcare, according to Danny McCormick of Harvard Medical School, the study's lead author.

The rates of preventable hospitalizations were practically the same in the first few years of the Massachusetts health reform. Jason Millman, writing in *The Washington Post,* observed:

"The landmark 2006 Massachusetts healthcare law that inspired the federal overhaul didn't lead to a reduction in unnecessary and costly hospitalizations, and it didn't make the healthcare system more fair for minority groups."

More evidence of the failure of ObamaCare comes from a new report from the National Alliance on Mental Illness. The report states, *"patients with mental illness are no better off under ObamaCare."*

Reasons for ObamaCare Failure

John C. Goodman, writing in *Forbes,* gives several reasons for the failures of ObamaCare noted above:

- **High deductibles** – Although more people have health insurance under ObamaCare, the deductibles they have to pay are so high that most people are paying the full price of the bill out of their own pockets. The average deductible for a bronze plan (least expensive) was $5,081 for an individual and $10,386 for a family. Silver plans had average deductibles of $2,907 for individuals and $6,078 for families. (These are about twice the average deductibles for employer plans.)
- **Medicaid poor access** – It is well known that patients with Medicaid coverage have poor access to healthcare because

few physicians accept these patients. Over 70 percent of newly enrolled patients in ObamaCare have Medicaid coverage.
- **Narrow networks** – By limiting the choice of physicians to narrow networks, insurance companies can lower the cost of premiums. Most ObamaCare plans offered on the exchanges have narrow networks. This has especially limited the choices of patients seeking mental illness treatments.

These alarming studies make a strong argument that *one year later with ObamaCare we are no better off than we were before!* ObamaCare is *not working.* We need a better alternative – and the sooner the better!

Some Liberals See the Light

Even the liberal media is beginning to see the reality of this nightmare. The *New Republic* admitted the launch of ObamaCare was "*a fiasco that could haunt progressives for years to come.*" They continued, "*Liberalism has spent the better part of the past century attempting to prove that it could competently and responsibly extend the state into new reaches of American life. With the rollout of the Affordable Care Act, the administration has badly injured that cause.*"

The failures of ObamaCare are not just the failures of President Obama and his administration. They are the failures of the Ruling Class in general. They are the failures of all those who believe that only the elite with proper credentials and social pedigree are qualified to lead this country.

Arguably the greatest president of the last fifty years, Ronald Reagan, was not a member of the Ruling Class. He was never respected by the intellectual elite and never given credit for his superior grasp of the world and its complexities. Yet he was the one whose tough foreign policy with the Soviet Union and strong national defense budget led to victory in the Cold War. His "supply-side economics" proved the Keynesians wrong and led to a great economic recovery.

Now every Republican, and even some liberals like Obama, tries to portray themself in the image of Reagan.

It wasn't supposed to be this way. Jonathan Chait, writing in *The New Republic,* founded by liberal progressive icon Herbert Croly, bragged on the Affordable Care Act when it was first passed. He opined:

"Historians will see this health care bill as a masterfully crafted piece of legislation. The new law untangles the dysfunctionalities of the individual insurance market while fulfilling the political imperative of leaving the employer-provided system in place. . . They put into place numerous reforms to force efficiency into a wasteful system. They found hundreds of billions of dollars in payment off-sets, a monumental task in itself. And they will bring economic and financial security to tens of millions of Americans who would otherwise risk seeing their lives torn apart."

But ObamaCare has done *none* of these things. Emery's conclusions are profound:

"It did not fix the dysfunctions of the individual market; it destroyed it. It did not save money; it squandered billions. It did not bring peace and security to tens of millions of people; it took it away from them. The best and the brightest had made their predictions. They were wrong."

Indeed, even some liberals are finally conceding this fundamental truth. Burke Beu, a life-long Democrat, Obama supporter and contributor, and a frequent volunteer for numerous Democratic candidates, confessed his disillusionment after the mid-term shellacking of the Democratic candidates. Mr. Beu, a nonprofit professional and former hospital insurance coordinator, is currently working as a counselor at a social-services agency in Denver.

In an Op-Ed published in *The Wall Street Journal* Beu writes:

"ObamaCare is a failure. For anyone who thinks this is a misprint because no Democratic activist would make such a comment, let me

add that it is too big, too complicated and too expensive. . . . It punishes responsible consumers like me and treats younger individuals as fools who are expected to pay the bills while not paying attention."

Then, in a testimonial that seems to come straight from the books of Codevilla and Siegel mentioned above, Beu makes this confessional:

"We (Democrats) say that we are the party of the people, but "the people" too often become a singular, monolithic concept for us. **We speak for the people, don't you know, because we can decide what is best for them so they really don't need to speak for themselves. The people decided otherwise on Election Day.** *I hope my party is listening. When the next Congress convenes in 2015, Democrats need to work with the new Republican majority, repeal ObamaCare, override a presidential veto if necessary, and start from scratch on health-care reform."*

Such great expectations – but so little achievement. It's amazing how ideology can blind one to *reality.* Thankfully, some like Mr. Beu are recognizing ObamaCare for the train wreck that Senator Max Baucus so famously predicted in April of 2013. His prediction has now become *The ObamaCare Reality.*

Dispelling the myths and documenting the reality of ObamaCare has been the purpose of this book. Those with open minds will be able to see the truth for what it is. Sadly, don't expect Progressives to give up their dream without a fight. A hundred years is a long time to wait.

Acknowledgements

Every author understands that writing is only half the battle. Getting published is the other crucial part of the process. For my start in the world of publishing, I am indebted to my literary agents, Sealy Yates and Mike Salisbury of Yates and Yates. Their professional expertise and guidance through the publication process were greatly appreciated. Their integrity and encouragement are priceless commodities in this fallen world.

Much appreciation is also given to the many friends, too numerous to mention, whose encouragement and affirmation have kept me motivated in the long hours of researching and writing this book. It is for good people like these that this book is written – that they might know the truth when the truth is in such short supply from our government. My hope is that this work has kept you informed and able to navigate the complexities of this new healthcare law – and encouraged you to pressure your Congressional representatives to improve it.

Lastly, I want to thank my family, especially my wife and my brother, for your encouragement, too. They have both been great affirmers of me. Her editorial touch has made this both readable and grammatically up to the standards of my early English teachers – and for that I am truly grateful. God bless you.

About the Author

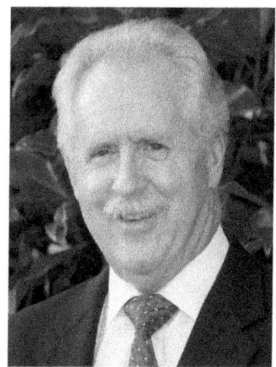

Robert S. Roberts, M.D. is an orthopedic surgeon still practicing medicine in Orlando, Florida. He is the author of *The ObamaCare Train Wreck,* which preceded this book and describes the historical record of the last 100 years of healthcare reform, the debate and passage of the Affordable Care Act and the early failures of the implementation of the law in 2013. This second book picks up where the first one ended in April, 2014, and traces the early months of the law's actual experience through the end of March, 2015.

Dr. Roberts writes a twice-weekly healthcare blog, called *Dr. Bob's ObamaCare Blog,* that can be found at www.drbobroberts.com. He also serves as a healthcare consultant to business and has been influential in promoting litigation that seeks relief from the provisions of ObamaCare that infringe upon religious liberty.

References

Introduction

1. *ObamaCare Fails to Fail* – Paul Krugman, *The New York Times,* 7/13/14
2. *Do Americans Dislike ObamaCare More Than Obama Likes Golf?* – Jeffery H. Anderson, *The Weekly Standard,* 8/26/14
3. *Democrats Against Reform* – Paul Krugman, *The New York Times,* 12/4/14

Chapter One – *The Premature Celebration*

1. *Kathleen Sebelius: Exchange enrollment goal is 7 million by end of March* – Jennifer Haberkorn, *Politico,* 6/24/13
2. *Sebelius Denies WH Ever Aimed for 7 Million Signups* – Wynton Hall, *Breitbart,* 2/25/14
3. *The ObamaCare Copperheads* – Editorial board, *The Wall Street Journal,* 4/1/14
4. *How Well Is ObamaCare Covering the Uninsured? A Glass Half Empty Moment* – Chris Conover, *Forbes,* 4/1/14
5. *ObamaCare Misses Its Target on the Uninsured by Half* – Jeffrey H. Anderson, *The Weekly Standard,* 7/15/14
6. *Last of the Broken Promises* – Robert S. Roberts, blog post www.drbobroberts.com, 6/29/14

7. *The Short Unhappy Life of ObamaCare* – Stephen Parente, *The Wall Street Journal*, 6/10/14

8. *Whatever Happened to Global Warming?* – Matt Ridley, *The Wall Street Journal*, 9/5/14

9. *QuickTake: Number of Uninsured Adults Continues to Fall under the ACA* – Urban Institute Policy Center, 7/10/14

10. *The "7.3 Million"* – Robert Laszewski, *Health Care Policy and Marketplace Review*, 9/19/14

11. *The ObamaCare Debate Is Far From Over* – Karl Rove, *The Wall Street Journal*, 4/10/14

Chapter Two – The Impact of Judicial Decisions

1. *The ObamaCare Train Wreck* – Robert S. Roberts, M.D. – Amazon, August 2014, Chapter 4

2. *The Pill Pettifoggery* - David Catron, The American Spectator, Jan-Feb 2014

3. *The Hobby Lobby Ruling* – John Daniel Davidson – *National Review Online*, 7/1/14

4. *Hobby Lobby Hysteria* –John McCormick, *The Weekly Standard*, 7/14/14

5. *After Hobby Lobby Comes Judge Pryor* – Quin Hillyer, *National Review Online*, 7/2/14

6. *Liberals Hobby Lobby Doublethink* –Jonah Goldberg, *National Review Online*, 7/2/14

7. *Administration Points to Hobby Lobby Ruling In Wheaton College Case* - Jess Bravin, *The Wall Street Journal*, 7/2/14

8. *ObamaCare's Latest Legal Challenge* – Editorial board, *The Wall Street Journal*, 3/23/14

9. *Get Ready for an Even Bigger Threat to ObamaCare* – Jonathan Turley, *Los Angeles Times*, 6/30/14

10. *ObamaCare's Biggest Legal Threat* – John Fund, *National Review Online*, 7/13/14

11. *ObamaCare Faces Another Court Threat – and This One Could Be Fatal* – Editorial Board, *The Wall Street Journal*, 7/7/14

12. *What the Supreme Court's Greenhouse Gas ruling Should Mean for ObamaCare* - Jeffrey Dorfman, *Forbes*, 6/24/14

13. *Decision Imminent in Case Challenging ObamaCare Subsidies* – Lucy Wescott, *Newsweek*, 7/7/14

14. *The ObamaCare – IRS Nexus* – Kimberley A. Strassel, *The Wall Street Journal*, 7/24/14

15. *Reining in ObamaCare – and the President* – Jonathan Adler and Michael F. Cannon, *The Wall Street Journal*, 7/23/14

16. *Upholding ObamaCare – as Written* – Editorial Board, *The Wall Street Journal*, 7/23/14

17. *Fast-Tracking ObamaCare to the Supremes* – Editorial Board, *The Wall Street Journal*, 7/23/14

18. *Why Democrats Packed the Court* – Editorial Board, *The Wall Street Journal*, 7/7/14

19. *Supreme Court Poised For a Do-Over on ObamaCare* – Chris Conover, *Forbes*, 9/30/14

20. *ObamaCare's Wonderland* – Editorial board, *The Wall Street Journal*, 10/1/14

21. *Judge: IRS ObamaCare Rule 'Is Arbitrary, Capricious, and Abuse of Discretion'* – Chris Bannister, *CNS News.com*, 10/2/14

22. *Pruitt v. Burwell: IRS's Illegal ObamaCare Taxes/Spending Suffer Another Defeat In Federal Court* – Michael F. Cannon, *Forbes*, 9/30/14

23. *ObamaCare's State of Crisis* – Adam J. White, *The Weekly Standard*, 11/24/14

24. *What the House ObamaCare Lawsuit and 'King v. Burwell' Have in Common* – Michael F. Cannon, *Forbes*, 11/21/14

Chapter Three – *Trampling the Constitution*

1. *Obama a Constitutional Law Professor?* – FactCheck.org, 3/28/08

2. *35 Changes to ObamaCare . . . So Far* - Tyler Hartsfield and Grace-Marie Turner, *The Galen Institute*, 2/10/14

3. *ObamaCare Versus Rule of Law* - Betsy McCaughey, *The American Spectator*, Dec. 2013

4. *Jonathan Turley Says, 'The Thing Speaks for Itself'* - Jeannie DeAngelis, *American Thinker*, 2/14/14

5. *ObamaCare Changes Are "Dangerous" Precedent, Lawyers Say* - Andrea Billups, *Newsmax*, 2/14/14

6. *myConstitution* - Jeffrey H. Anderson, *The Weekly Standard*, 2/10/14

7. *ObamaCare Lawlessness Charge Sticks* - Jennifer Rubin, *The Washington Post*, 2/12/14

8. *Extension Expected on Health Policies Not Meeting Law* - Louise Radnofsky and Anna Wilde Mathews, *The Wall Street Journal*, 3/4/14

9. *ObamaCare: 'Obviously Inadmissible'* - Louie Gohmert & Joseph E. Schmitz, *National Review Online*, 3/3/14

10. *Obama Gives Health Plans Added Two-Year Reprieve* - Louis Radnofsky, *The Wall Street Journal*, 3/5/14

11. *Upholding the Law* - Jeff Bergner, *The Weekly Standard*, 3/10/14

12. *The Endangered Senators Rule* - Editorial, *The Wall Street Journal*, 3/5/14

13. *The Structure of the Government Must Furnish the Proper Checks and Balances Between the Different Departments* - James Madison, *Federalist 51*, 2/6/1788

14. *ObamaCare's Secret Mandate Exemption* - Editorial, *The Wall Street Journal*, 3/12/14

15. *ObamaCare's Latest Legal Challenge* - Editorial, *The Wall Street Journal*, 3/24/14

16. *42 Changes to ObamaCare . . . So Far* – Tyler Hartsfield and Grace-Marie Turner, *The Galen Institute*, 7/18/14

17. *The Gridlock Clause* – Josh Blackman, *National Review*, 9/8/14

18. *EEOC v. Hosanna-Tabor Evangelical Lutheran Church and School* – The Becket Fund.org, 1/11/12
19. *Obama's Enforcer* – John Fund and Hans von Spakovsky, Broadside Books, 2014

Chapter Four – *The Reality of Medicaid*

1. *On Schools, Taxes, Beer, Give 'em Hugs – or Give 'em Hell* – Scott Maxwell, *The Orlando Sentinel*, 4/13/14
2. *Why Medicaid is a Humanitarian Catastrophe* – Avik Roy, *Forbes*, 3/2/11
3. *How Medicaid Harms the Poor: A Counter-Rebuttal, Part I* – Avik Roy, *Forbes*, 3/9/11
4. *How Medicaid Harms the Poor: A Counter-Rebuttal, Part II* – Avik Roy, *Forbes*, 3/10/11
5. *How Medicaid Harms the Poor: A Counter-Rebuttal, Part III* – Avik Roy, *Forbes*, 3/11/11
6. *Priceless* – John H. Goodman, *The Independent Institute*, 2012
7. *Impact of Medicaid Expansion on Hospitals*: Updated for Second Quarter 2014 – Colorado Hospital Association, September 2014
8. *Visits to Emergency Departments Increased Three Times Faster in States That Expanded Medicaid Than Those That Did Not* – John R. Graham, *The National Center for Policy Analysis*, 9/10/14
9. *Better Healthcare for the Poor* –_Joseph R. Antos, James C. Capretta, Robert Doar, and Mark Pauly, *The Hill*, 5/20/14
10. *A Republican Victory on the Front Lines of ObamaCare* - Fred Barnes, *The Wall Street Journal*, 7/11/14
11. *A Regional Assessment of Medicaid Access to Outpatient Orthopaedic Care* –_Patterson, Draeger, Olsson, Spang, Lin, and Kamath, *The Journal of Bone and Joint Surgery*, 9/17/14
12. *ObamaCare: Fewer Doctors, More Demand* – Michael Tanner, *National Review Online*, 9/10/14

Chapter Five – *The Insurance Bailout Has Begun*

1. *Bailing Out Health Insurers and Helping ObamaCare* – Jeffrey H. Anderson, *The Weekly Standard,* 1/13/14
2. *The Slush Fund* – Jay Cost and Jeffrey H. Anderson, *The Weekly Standard,* 5/12/14
3. *ObamaCare Insurer Subsidies in Action: The Case of Humana* – Jay Cost, *The Weekly Standard,* 5/8/14
4. *The White House is Bribing Health Insurance Companies* – Avik Roy, *Forbes,* 7/14/14
5. *An Unfolding Fiscal Disaster* – Charles Blahous, *The Weekly Standard,* 7/14/14
6. *Sink the ObamaCare Bailout* – Deroy Murdock, *National Review Online,* 8/27/14
7. *Laszewski, Back From Summer Vacation, Still Predicts ObamaCare Train Wreck* – John R. Graham, *National Center for Policy Analysis,* 9/8/14
8. *The Next Chapter of ObamaCare* – Robert Laszewski, *Health Care Policy and Marketplace Review,* 9/7/14
9. *Don't Take a Knee, GOP* – Jeffrey H. Anderson, *The Weekly Standard,* 9/15/14
10. *ObamaCare and American Decline* – Holman W. Jenkins, Jr., *The Wall Street Journal,* 9/16/14

Chapter Six – *Socialized Medicine*

1. *Where ObamaCare is Going* – Scott W. Atlas, *The Wall Street Journal,* 8/14/14
2. *What Sweden Can Teach Us About ObamaCare* – Per Bylund, *The Wall Street Journal,* 4/18/14
3. *Mirror, Mirror on the Wall, 2014 Update: How the U.S. Health Care System Compares Internationally* – Executive Summary, *The Commonwealth Fund*

4. *ObamaCare: The Plan is to Transition to "Single-Payer" Socialized Medicine* – William F. Jasper, *The New American,* 11/8/13

5. *Health Care is Moving Toward a Single-Payer System* – Douglas W. Jackson, *Orthopedics Today,* April 2013

6. *British Experience with NHS Reveals Ills of Government Health Care Programs Like ObamaCare* – Cal Thomas, *The Washington Examiner,* 1/15/14

7. *Britain's NHS Seeks to Limit Care for Smokers and Obese Individuals* – Kenneth Artz, *Heartland Institute,* 5/13/11

8. *What ObamaCare Can Learn From Britain's National Health Service* – John C. Goodman, *National Center for Policy Analysis,* 10/10/13

9. *Canada's ObamaCare Precedent* – David Gratzer, *The Wall Street Journal,* 6/9/09

10. *If Universal Health Care is the Goal, Don't Copy Canada* – Jason Clemens and Bacchus Barua, *Forbes,* 6/13/14

11. *A Look Into Canadian Health Care* – National Center for Policy Analysis, 10/17/13

12. *The Effect of Wait Times on Mortality in Canada* – Nadeem Esmail, *The Fraser Institute,* 5/20/14

13. *Single-Payer National Health Insurance Around the World* – Ch. 2 – Goodman, Musgrave, and Herrick, Rowman and Littlefield Publishers, 2004

14. *Private Healthcare: the Lessons From Sweden* – Randeep Ramesh, *The Guardian,* 12/18/12

15. *What Sweden Teaches Us About ObamaCare* – National Center for Policy Analysis, 4/24/14

16. *Swiss Health Care: The Good, The Bad, and The Ugly* – John C. Goodman, Healthblog.ncpa.org, 10/19/09

17. *Taking the Government Out of Health Care* – National Center for Policy Analysis, 9/8/14

18. *U.S. Has the Worst Health Care? Not By a Long Shot* – Sally Pipes, *Forbes,* 7/14/14

19. *Single-Payer National Health Insurance Around the World – Ch. 8* – Goodman, Musgrave, and Herrick, Rowman and Littlefield Publishers, 2004
20. *Don't Just Replace ObamaCare – Replace the Great Society* – Avik Roy, *The Weekly Standard*, 9/4/14

Chapter Seven – *The VA Scandal*

1. *About VA* – U.S. Department of Veterans Affairs, www.va.gov, 9/29/14
2. *Doctors' War Stories From VA Hospitals* – Hal Scherz, *The Wall Street Journal*, 5/28/14
3. *No, The VA Isn't a Preview of ObamaCare – It's Much Worse* – Avik Roy, *Forbes*, 5/23/14
4. *Confessions of a Whistleblower* – Brian Mockenhaupt, *AARP Bulletin*, Sept 2014
5. *VA Scandal Shows How Government Works* – Jeffrey Dorfman, *Forbes*, 5/24/14
6. *Does the VA Scandal Make 'ObamaCare' Look Bad?* – Napp Nazworth, *The Christian Post*, 5/27/14
7. *The VA Scandal's Lesson for ObamaCare* – Editorial board, *New York Post*, 5/21/14
8. *Real Accountability at the VA* – Editorial board, *The Wall Street Journal*, 5/31/14
9. *The VA's Bonus Culture* – Editorial board, *The Wall Street Journal*, 5/30/14
10. *Big Labor's VA Choke Hold* – Kimberley Strassel, *The Wall Street Journal*, 5/30/14
11. *The VA Scandal is a Crisis of Leadership* – Peggy Noonan, *The Wall Street Journal*, 5/31/14
12. *The Government Health-Care Model* – Editorial board, *The Wall Street Journal*, 5/23/14
13. *The Real VA Problem* – Mark Hemingway, *The Weekly Standard*, 6/9/14

14. *Restoring Trust in VA Health Care* – Kenneth W. Kizer and Ashish K. Jha, *New England Journal of Medicine*, 6/4/14
15. *Political Triage at the VA* – Editorial board, *The Wall Street Journal*, 6/7/14
16. *The Second VA Scandal* – Editorial board, *The Wall Street Journal*, 6/19/14
17. *Beyond the Waiting Lists, New Senate Report Reveals a Culture of Crime, Cover-up and Coercion Within the VA* – Senator Tom Coburn, Press release, 6/24/14

Chapter Eight – *The Abortion Reality*

1. *GAO Report Shows How ObamaCare Subsidizes Abortion* – Timothy P. Carney, *The Washington Examiner*, 9/15/14
2. *Three Ways ObamaCare Forces Americans to Fund Big Abortion* – Casey Mattox, *The Federalist*, 9/23/14
3. *ObamaCare's Taxpayer-Funded Abortions* – Carl Anderson, *National Review Online*, 9/17/14
4. *ObamaCare's Abortion Shell Game* – Arina O. Grossu, *National Review Online*, 9/15/14
5. *ObamaCare Forcing Pro-Life Family to Pay for Other People's Abortions* – Casey Mattox and Matt Bowman, *Alliance Defending Freedom*, 5/2/14
6. *ObamaCare Funds Abortions* – Robert S. Roberts, *Dr. Bob's Healthcare Blog*, 10/6/14
7. *House Bans ObamaCare Subsidies for Abortion Coverage* – Paige Winfield Cunningham, *Politico*, 1/28/14
8. *House Passes Bill to Ban Abortions From Being Covered Under ObamaCare* – Fox News, Associated Press, 1/28/14
9. *Stupak, Dems Reach Abortion Deal,* - Jared Allen and Jeffrey Young, *The Hill*, 3/21/10
10. *H.R. 7: No Taxpayer Funding for Abortion and Abortion Insurance Full Disclosure Act of 2014* – Library of Congress, 1/28/14

Chapter Nine – *The Cost of ObamaCare – Economic Reality*

9. *Has the Affordable Care Act Slowed the Growth of Health Care Spending?* – Andrew J. Rettenmaier, Thomas R. Saving, and Zijun Wang, *National Center for Policy Analysis*, 7/23/14

10. *Medical Mergers Are Driving Up Health Costs* – Suzanne F. Delbanco, *The Wall Street Journal*, 9/30/14

11. *The Unfolding Fiscal Disaster Behind ACA Enrollment Figures* – Charles Blahous, *Mercatus Center – George Mason University*, 4/17/14

12. *An Unfolding Fiscal Disaster* – Charles Blahous, *The Weekly Standard*, 7/14/14

13. *ObamaCare's Failing Cost Control* – Editorial board, *The Wall Street Journal*, 10/20/14

14. *Now There Can Be No Doubt: ObamaCare Has Increased Non-group Premiums in Nearly All States* – Chris Conover, *Forbes*, 10/23/14

Chapter Ten – *The Impact on Jobs and Innovation*

1. *What Happens to the Unemployment Rate If You Add Back Labor Force Dropouts?* – Sean Davis, *Economics*, 5/2/14

2. *Say Hello to the GOP's New Favorite Statistic: Workforce Participation* – Jordan Weissmann, *The Atlantic*, 2014

3. *Don't Be Fooled, The Obama Unemployment Rate is 11%* - Peter Ferrara, *Forbes*, 2/9/12

4. *Why Can't People Find a Job? One Big Reason is ObamaCare* – John C. Goodman, *Forbes*, 8/25/14

5. *How ObamaCare's Employer Mandate Harms Low-Wage Workers* – Rep. Bill Cassidy and Chase Lindsey, *Forbes*, 9/17/14

6. *ObamaCare is Dampening the Job Market in 3 Principal Ways* – Avik Roy, *Forbes*, 9/1/14

7. *Wal-Mart to End Health Insurance for Some Part-Time Employees* – Shelly Banjo, Anna Wilde Mathews, and Theo Francis, *The Wall Street Journal*, 10/7/14

8. *Everyday Low Benefits* – The Editorial board, *The Wall Street Journal*, 10/7/14

9. *ObamaCare's Anti-Innovation Effect* – Scott W. Atlas, *The Wall Street Journal,* 10/1/14

10. *ObamaCare: Sending Research, Development and Innovation Overseas* – *National Center for Policy Analysis, 10/6/14*

11. *Part-Time Employees May Be Better Off Under ObamaCare than full-Time Workers* – *National Center for Policy Analysis*, 10/10/14

12. *The Affordable Care Act and the New Economics of Part-time Work* – Casey Mulligan, *Mercatus Center,* 10/7/14

Chapter Eleven – *ObamaCare and Income Inequality*

1. *Income Inequality and Rising Health-Care Costs* – Mark J. Warshawsky and Andrew G. Biggs, *The Wall Street Journal,* 10/6/14

2. *How ObamaCare Will Fuel Income Inequality in the U.S.* – Chris Conover, *Forbes, 9/11/14*

3. *The President of Inequality* –Editorial board, *The Wall Street Journal,* 10/2/14

4. *Minimum Wage, Maximum Politics* – Andy Puzder, *The Wall Street Journal,* 10/5/14

5. *Minimum Wage Backfire* – Editorial board, *The Wall Street Journal,* 10/22/14

6. *The Gelded Age* – Kevin D. Williamson, *National Review Online,* 9/30/14

7. *The Minimum-Wage Stealth Tax on the Poor* – Thomas Macurdy, *The Wall Street Journal,* 2/22/15

8. *The Unappetizing Effect of Minimum-Wage Hikes* – Michael Saltsman, *The Wall Street Journal,* 3/25/15

Chapter Twelve – *Alternatives That Work*

1. *The Economics of Replacing ObamaCare: The Good, The Bad, and The Ugly* – Peter Ferrara, *Forbes, 6/1/14*

2. *Hitting the Political Sweetspot on an ObamaCare Alternative –* James C. Capretta and Jeffrey H. Anderson, *The Weekly Standard,* 6/5/14

3. *Here Are Good ways to Replace ObamaCare, Not Simply Repeal It –* James C. Capretta, *The Washington Examiner,* 6/20/14

4. *A Winning Alternative to ObamaCare –* The 2017 Project, *2017Project.org*

5. *Scoring of the 2017 Project's 'Winning Alternative to ObamaCare'* – Jeffrey H. Anderson, *2017Project.org,* 9/8/14

6. *Getting There – How to Transition From ObamaCare to Real Health Care Reform –* James C. Capretta and Yuval Levin, *The Weekly Standard,* 9/22/14

7. *Transcending ObamaCare: An Introduction to Patient-Centered, Consumer-Driven Health Reform –* Avik Roy, *Forbes,* 8/13/14

8. *Transcending ObamaCare: A Patient-Centered Plan for Near-Universal Coverage and Permanent Fiscal Solvency –* Avik Roy, *Manhattan Institute for Policy Research,* August 2014

9. *Replacing ObamaCare Saves a Lot of Money –* James C. Capretta, *National Review Online,* 9/19/14

10. *2017 Project's Alternative to ObamaCare Gets a Boost –* William Kristol, *The Weekly Standard,* 9/8/14

11. *An ObamaCare Do-Over –* Ed Gillespie, *The New York Times,* 11/20/14

12. *The Impressive new ObamaCare Replace Plan From Republicans Burr, Hatch, and Upton –* Avik Roy, *Forbes,* 2/5/15

13. *GOP Proposal Scraps Taxes, Opens Choice, Retains Continuous Coverage –* Orrin Hatch, Fred Upton, and Richard Burr – *USA Today,* 2/5/15

Chapter Thirteen – *The Future of Medicare*

1. *The Independent Payment Advisory Board – PPACA's Anti-Constitutional and Authoritarian Super-Legislature –* Diane Cohen and Michael F. Cannon, *The Cato Institute,* 6/14/12

2. *Medicare Cuts Under ObamaCare Will Affect Low-Income Seniors Most* – National Center for Policy Analysis, 3/13/13
3. *Healthcare for the Poor, or Poor Healthcare?* – Joseph Antos, *Real Clear Markets*, 3/6/13
4. *What Seniors Have to Fear From ObamaCare* – John C. Goodman, *Forbes*, 10/28/14
5. *Fixing the Doc Fix* – National Center for Policy Analysis, 10/28/14
6. *Doc Fix Problems and Solutions* – Hadley Manning, *Independent Women's Forum*, November 2014
7. *ObamaCare vs. Medicare* – Jeffrey H. Anderson, *The Weekly Standard*, 3/10/14
8. *Press Release: Trustees Report Shows Continued Reduced Cost Growth, Longer Medicare Solvency* – CMS.gov, 7/28/14
9. *Medicare Hype* – John C. Goodman, *Forbes*, 7/29/14
10. *The New York Times is Wrong: Medicare is Still a Budget Buster* – Chris Conover, *Forbes*, 8/31/14
11. *Romney vs. Obama: The Romney-Ryan Medicare Plan Compared to the Obama Medicare Plan – Who's Telling the Truth?* – Robert Laszewski, *Health Care Policy and Marketplace Review*, 8/20/12
12. *Jeanne Shaheen's Dishonest Claim That ObamaCare Doesn't Cut Medicare* – Avik Roy, *Forbes*, 10/22/14
13. *ObamaCare: Fewer Doctors, More Demand* – Michael Tanner, *National Review Online*, 9/10/14

Chapter Fourteen – *The Gruber Tapes*

1. *The Gruber Confession* – Charles Krauthammer, *National Review Online*, 11/13/14
2. *Gruber Who?* – Ian Tuttle, *National Review Online*, 11/14/14
3. *Jonathan Gruber's 'Stupid' Budget Tricks* – Editorial Board, *The Wall Street Journal*, 11/14/14
4. *Gruber Is Also Wrong On Policy* - Grace-Marie Turner, *Forbes*, 11/13/14

5. *ACA Architect: 'The Stupidity of the American Voter' Led Us to Hide ObamaCare's True Costs From the Public* – Avik Roy, *Forbes,* 11/10/14

6. *Two More Gruber Videos: ObamaCare Architect Boasts of Law's 'Exploitation' of the American Voter* – Avik Roy, *Forbes,* 11/13/14

7. *Another ObamaCare Deception* - Tevi Troy, *The Wall Street Journal,* 11/16/14

8. *White House Disagrees With 'Stupidity' Remarks* - Justin Sink, *The Hill,* 11/13/14

9. *Academic Built Case for Mandate in Health Care Law* - Catherine Rampell, *The New York Times,* 3/28/12

10. *Thank You, Jonathan Gruber* - Rich Lowry, *National Review Online,* 11/14/14

11. *GOP's Anti-ObamaCare Push Gains New Momentum in Wake of Gruber Video* – Robert Costa and Jose A. DelReal, *The Washington Post,* 11/12/14

Chapter Fifteen – *The Impact of the Mid-Term Elections*

1. *Seven ObamaCare bills That the New GOP Senate Majority Should Pass in 2015* – Avik Roy, *Forbes,* 11/5/14

2. *Republican Wave Put ObamaCare in Surgery, and These Parts Could Be Amputated* – Scott Gottlieb, *Forbes,* 11/10/14

3. *Now Can We Finally "Wave" Goodbye to ObamaCare?* – Chris Conover, *Forbes,* 11/11/14

4. *Greatest Builder of the Republican Party Since Ronald Reagan* – George Will, *Fox News Special Report,* 11/19/14

5. *ObamaCare's Twilight: health Reform in the Next Congress* – John R. Graham and Devon Herrick, *Forbes* and *National Center for Policy Analysis,* 11/5/14

6. *Repeal, And Replace, The Employer Mandate* – Timothy Jost, *Health Affairs Blog,* 6/4/14

7. *From Success to Success,* - Jay Cost, *The Weekly Standard,* 11/17/14

Chapter Sixteen – *Conclusions*